Migraine Relief with HYPNOSIS

Advance Praise

"This book explains how hypnosis works and specifically why it is helpful for migraine headaches. The author describes her own lifelong history of migraine pain, and how hypnosis helped her. She was a nurse before she became a hypnotist and her knowledgeable and caring manner comes right through in her writing. I felt like she was talking directly to me. I highly recommend this book. This book does such a good job of describing hypnosis from the perspective of the client and from the perspective of the hypnotist that it would be useful for anyone considering hypnosis for any problem, not just migraine pain."

– Tamara Sterling

"The author has a gentle and affirming style—establishing rapport quickly with the reader by explaining what's in store and sharing her personal experiences to put the reader at ease and help them feel not quite so alone in their suffering. I was so impressed by the holistic, flowing quality of the book. Kathie skillfully leads the reader into the heart of the hypnosis experience, inviting them to look inside for answers, introducing important topics in easy-to-understand language, and providing useful resources and techniques to help the reader feel empowered and achieve success. Her focus on self-compassion, the vital role of forgiveness, and the importance of practicing the recommended techniques all provide readers with a very effective program for achieving relief from migraine headaches and for making other key positive life changes in the process. Thank you for taking the time to write this remarkable healing resource!"

– **Stephe Newell Niggemeyer**

"In *Migraine Relief with Hypnosis* Kathie Hardy provides hope to those experiencing migraines, along with a path to overcome them with hypnosis. Kathie weaves her own journey with migraines along with a detailed explanation of how hypnosis can help- both through her own story as well as through an excellent explanation of hypnotic techniques that have been proven to help many others with migraines as well as other issues."

– **Brenda Titus**

"This new book is a gem of details, not only just on the dreaded headaches, but on a variety of solutions, for general health and well-being, with and without hypnosis. I am very impressed and recommend this book to anyone who has—or knows someone who suffers from—the pain of migraines, or needs to know more about how hypnosis can help."

– **Lynne Potter Lord**

"With Kathie's years of expertise in the medical field, combined with her knowledge of hypnosis and loving nature she provides hope in her book to the many that have not been able to find relief from the overwhelming grip of migraine pain. As a former migraine sufferer, I found *Migraine Relief with Hypnosis* a light in the dark as she explains this alternative to pharmaceutical treatment."

– Amanda Troy

"Kathie is an amazing hypnotist, not only because she is compassionate and kind, but because she has a lifetime of experience to draw from. Her time being a registered nurse helped her see what was and was not possible in the field she worked in for so many years. She is dedicated to being current on all that hypnosis has to offer the modern-day practitioner and she spends a lot of time keeping her education and knowledge up to date. As her book states she suffered for years from debilitating migraine headaches and she tried everything she could to alleviate her problem. This book will change your life, it will make a difference in ways you never imagined. Kathie explains hypnosis and how it can help you in a way that is very easy to understand and easy to accept. If you suffer from any kind of debilitating pain or physical symptoms that prevent you from living your best life, this book is where you need to start to get your life back!"

– Paulette Deckers

"Being a once migraine suffer myself, Kathie has presented very informative facts and materials that will truly help with migraine relief. I personally received relief from the 7th Path Self-Hypnosis® process and can attest that the suggestions of the author are factual and helpful. This is a quick and informative read. You will NOT be disappointed."

– Marcella Hilferty

"Reading this book I found another way to help friends and family deal with their migraine issues. Kathie presents the information in an easy to understand way."

– Denise Aguilar

Migraine Relief with HYPNOSIS

*How a Few Minutes Every Day Can Give You
Energy, Clarity, and Enthusiasm to
Take Care of Yourself and Your Family*

Katherine Hardy

NEW YORK

LONDON • NASHVILLE • MELBOURNE • VANCOUVER

Migraine Relief with HYPNOSIS
*How a Few Minutes Every Day Can Give You Energy, Clarity,
and Enthusiasm to Take Care of Yourself and Your Family*

© 2020 Katherine Hardy

Published in New York, New York, by Morgan James Publishing in partnership with Difference Press. Morgan James is a trademark of Morgan James, LLC.
www.MorganJamesPublishing.com

Disclaimer
Pain is an important signal from your body that something may be wrong. I require a referral from a physician before helping clients with pain management using hypnosis. Once your doctor has determined that anything potentially dangerous has been ruled out and there is nothing more he or she can do, then come see me. Then it is safe and ethical for me to help you reduce or eliminate pain. Hypnosis is safe, effective, and has no negative side effects.

Client names have been changed to respect privacy.

ISBN 978-1-64279-679-7 paperback
ISBN 978-1-64279-680-3 eBook
ISBN 978-1-64279-681-0 audio
Library of Congress Control Number: 2019907381

Cover Design by:
Chris Treccani
www.3dogcreative.net

Interior Design by:
Bonnie Bushman
The Whole Caboodle Graphic Design

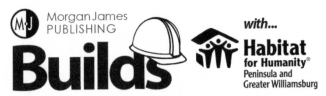

Morgan James is a proud partner of Habitat for Humanity Peninsula and Greater Williamsburg. Partners in building since 2006.

Get involved today! Visit
www.MorganJamesBuilds.com

For anyone who has ever felt the severe pain of
a migraine headache coming on and thought,
Oh, no, not again!
This book is for you.

Table of Contents

Introduction

You've got a book in your hands about hypnosis helping with migraine pain. My guess is you have already been suffering from migraine headaches for some time. Buying a book means you are really ready to hear some new ideas and take some new action. You want something in your life to change. Migraine pain and conventional medical treatments are complicated. Last I checked, there were fifty-three medications commonly prescribed for migraines. Many of them work very well, and all of them work for someone. Despite my nursing background, I am not going to discuss the pros and cons of medications, and I am not going to give you a pile of statistics to wade through. Information like that is readily available via Google. And besides, statistics are not going to change anything for you right now. You know clearly what you want. Less pain. No pain would be even better. And I'm not going to do more than mention here how the opioid addiction crisis is having an enormous impact on our society and causing untold suffering in the lives of people who become addicted in their understandable desire to be pain-free. Often, difficulties in life are accompanied by loneliness and a feeling of isolation. You have been struggling for a long time.

I'm going to tell you how I was helped, after decades of pain. There are multiple triggers for every person who suffers from migraine headaches. Everyone's experience is different. There are things you can do on your own that may be helpful. I'll remind you of external triggers which you can manage to one degree or another, like environmental exposure, food, dehydration, your own hormonal fluctuations. And there's hypnosis for the parts that are hard to get to, the deep personal sources of stress.

I suffered for forty-six years. I tried all the things I'm going to remind you to try, and some of them did help. Note what helps you, and do it. Cast a wide net. Use everything you can to keep yourself comfortable. I tried everything I could before I stumbled on hypnosis. And for me, hypnosis made all the difference. I hope it helps you.

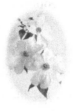

Chapter 1

Migraines Are
Stealing Your Life

Migraines steal your life from you. You've had head-aches for longer than you can remember. People who don't have headaches can't even relate. There are some people who have never had a headache in their lives. What would that be like? You've tried everything, and nothing has worked, or some things seemed to work for a while and before you knew it, you were waking up again to that vise-grip of pain. Or maybe it was a deep dull ache accompanied by photophobia, and you couldn't stand any light in your eyes. Maybe you found yourself on the edge of vomiting from the pain. Or you *were* vomiting. Whatever your experience, you are one of millions of people in the U.S. alone who suffer from migraine headache pain. People all over the world suffer. The World Health Organization ranks migraine as one of the top 20 causes of years of healthy life lost to disability. And it's not just the pain, the light sensitivity, the nausea. It's also the anticipation, the dread of pain, the fear—fear because you know you're in for hours of discomfort at best and incapacitation from pain at worst. Headaches derail your plans for the day and complicate the following days as a result. They have a nasty habit of occurring just when something important is happening in your life, just when you need all your mental and emotional energy. Wham! there's a migraine. A "sick headache" they used to call them in the olden days.

You have missed events in your life. You've probably let your family down, your partner down, your kids down, your friends down, your workplace down, maybe even your pets down. No dog is getting a long ball session with an owner in the grip of a migraine.

You have missed family breakfasts, special dinners, celebrations. You have missed parts of the holidays. Other people have had to carry your load because of your migraines—housekeeping didn't get done. There are vacations you never got to take, and that perhaps your *family* didn't get to take because you used all your time off from work being sick. Beyond that, there's getting the kids off to school or transporting them to after-school soccer practice, attending scout meetings, and even people picking up your load at work. No one likes to work with someone who calls in sick all the time. Your partner may even have had to take time off work to do the things you were going to do that day if they involved caring for children or other family members. You have let yourself down because you haven't figured out how to get out from under the weight of this pain.

It's not just the sheer pain and the dread of pain. The *memory* of pain is stressful, as well as the *regret* about missing out on things. All the things you didn't do when you were in the midst of a headache either got done by someone else— and there is a cost to that—or they are still waiting for you to do them, but now you have fewer hours in your day in which to do them. It feels like a lose-lose situation no matter how you look at it. It sucks. Migraines are time-sucking, energy-sucking, enthusiasm-sucking, dream-sucking, *life*-sucking problems.

Not solving your migraine problem is expensive. In business school terms, there is a "lost opportunity cost"—all the opportunities for all the shared experiences you've missed, the meetings you've missed. All the things you couldn't do because you were busy having a migraine.

Treating your migraines with medications adds another layer of problems all on their own. You have to see a doctor usually more than once, you have to pick them up at a pharmacy, you have to pay for them, and even if you have insurance, there is nearly always a copay. And all medications have side effects. *And* you have to go through this effort whether or not the migraine medications work. The process of evaluating several medications to see which one works can take months. Once you finally have a prescription for one that works for you, it might take two hours to work each time. Two hours is a long time when you are having so much pain you feel like you might throw up, and you can't get out of bed, or if you do manage to stand up, you have to keep the shades drawn and most of the lights off so you can tolerate having your eyes open. Even if you are able to pull yourself out of bed and get your kids off to school, that's a miserable way to live.

Then there's the Herculean effort of trying to figure out what *your* triggers are for migraines. Anyone who has ever had a migraine has put effort into trying to figure out what the cause was. What happened in the twelve hours before a migraine? What happened so we can make sure it *never* happens again? But it does happen again. And again. And again. It might be something basic and simple, like MSG—every time you go to a Chinese Restaurant where they use MSG you get a migraine. Lucky you, if that was all the detective work required to diagnose the source of your headaches. For most people, if MSG sensitivity is an issue for them, if they get a migraine every single time they eat at a Chinese restaurant, they can avoid Chinese restaurants and *still* have lots of migraines. There are other unknown triggers or causes of migraines.

Then there is the slippery slope of opioids. As a nurse, I have heard hundreds of patients relay stories about having some kind of chronic or recurring pain that did not get adequately treated, that resulted in a dependency on some sort of opioid medication—frequently Vicodin or oxycodone, or street drugs like meth or heroin. And opioid dependency is a hell all of its own—worrying about how and where to get enough, of course the inconvenience of having procurement be part of your everyday life—doctor appointments, pharmacy pickups, budgeting the money, keeping it away from children, (for some people, keeping it from getting stolen), or finding it on the street and risking drug charges in the legal system. There is the fear of, and the real experience of, being judged for not being "strong" enough, for not being able to "get over" your pain, for perhaps not following through with instructions to rest after a painful injury or with physical therapy homework. There are the labels of "drug seeking," "addicted," or "dependent," with the unspoken labels of "weak, lazy, stupid." There is a risk of getting a DUI if you drive while taking opioids. There is a risk of losing your job if your job includes drug tests or the possibility of making serious errors and being forced to take a drug test as part of the follow up investigation. And on the distant horizon, the shadow of knowing that some people lie to doctors and use multiple pharmacies with cash to get enough opioids to escape pain, or even worse, resort to street drugs and illegal activity, and that this could conceivably happen to you.

You lose hours and minutes that add up to days and weeks from migraine pain. And you don't get those hours and minutes back. If you have chronic migraines, loosely defined as more than fifteen migraines a month—that's the equivalent of *half* your days with migraine pain—then you are losing up to two hours every time you have a migraine. Of course, it's more than that because insurance companies, doctors, and pharmacists don't want you to have more than nine Imitrex tablets in a month, because of the risk of "rebound headaches"—a situation where you have a headache, take Imitrex, and then it swings you into another headache the following day (which maybe you wouldn't have had if you had just suffered until it finally went away, which could take days, or if you took two oxycodone tablets. This is just my personal example, remember there are fifty-two other medications.)

So nine days a month, you take Imitrex and lose two hours—that's eighteen hours—and perhaps three days that month, you take oxycodone and lose two hours—that's six hours plus the eighteen, totaling twenty-two, then add the three eight hour days when you just slogged through with no quality of life by extra caffeine and big doses of Tylenol or ibuprofen. Add those horrible twenty-four hours to the previous twenty-two, and you've got forty-six hours lost. Forty-six hours in one month.

But on the conservative side, if you only have fifteen migraines, each of which was treated with medication with a two hour wait time—that still means thirty hours every month.

Imagine what you could do with an extra thirty hours a month. You could learn to play an instrument, learn a foreign language, learn woodworking, golf, learn how to draw or paint. You could spend it with someone you love. You could take a couple of classes and advance your career. You could put in a garden, learn to swing dance. You could read some interesting books. But you are not doing any of these things during your thirty hours a month. You suffer from migraines.

It's not your fault that what you've tried isn't working. You probably deserve a medal for the detective work you've done on your life, for the hours you've spent trying to solve this problem.

I used to have migraines all the time. When I think back and add up all the hours I've spent in pain, I feel like crying. So much loss. So I know a little about what you are going through. I was you—but not anymore.

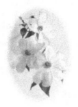

Chapter 2

My Story

It was Day Five of waking up at three am with a splitting vise-like headache. I was in a deep well of pain and I couldn't get out. A feeling of certainly flooded through me that it would be better to be dead than to continue to suffer like this. I felt panicky and resigned at the same time. I couldn't get away from the pain. I could hardly see. It hurt to open my eyes. Nausea filled my chest and throat. I'd taken Imitrex tablets on Days One, Two and Three when the pain woke me up each morning at three am. I wasn't supposed to take them more than three days in a row—concern about

9

rebound headaches, my doctor and my pharmacist said. The fourth day I took one oxycodone and finally got back to sleep. It didn't take the pain completely away, so I took big doses of Tylenol and ibuprofen and loaded up on caffeine. The pain receded slightly. I went to work and slogged through the day, knee deep in discomfort and feeling depressed. Today, Day Five, I would take another Imitrex. In two hours I knew I would feel better. But what about tomorrow? I didn't have enough of either drug to make it through the month. I thought, "I cannot live like this."

It's exhausting to be suicidal from pain. And now on top of the pain, on top of the anxiety about how to get pain relief, how to get the drugs I needed, how to not get addicted to opioids, is the layer of worry and stress from thinking about killing myself. My family– what I needed to do to make sure they were cared for, and figuring out a plan that would be effective and not leave me a vegetable on a ventilator. Guilt and more anxiety piled onto the mountain of emotions. I knew I couldn't keep living like this.

I went back to my doctor. She referred me to a nutritionist. I referred myself to a massage therapist, started seeing a chiropractor again, saw a cranial sacral therapist suggested by a friend. I cast a wide net—in subsequent months, I saw a neurologist. She tried Botox—just inside my hairline. It didn't work for my headaches, and it was in the wrong spot to help with wrinkles. I learned there was a pain clinic and got a referral and had a two-hour admission interview which was encouraging because the doctor seemed to know a great deal about pain. I spent six weeks recording everything I did, every single thing I ate. At the conclusion, I realized there were about twenty things that contributed to my headaches and I learned that I was just going to have to accept them and manage them. He put me on over-the-counter anti-inflammatory medications to help prevent the headaches, and reiterated the importance of not taking Imitrex more than three days in a row. I resigned myself to the fact that migraines were something I would have to manage my whole life.

Then I met a man on a ski lift at Mt. Baker who told me his wife had gotten relief from her headaches from a Chinese medicine doctor in Vancouver, B.C. Vancouver was closer to my home than Seattle, so the next week I drove over the border into Canada, and saw him. It was an adventure just walking through the enormous Asian market to get to his office, which was next to a Chinese apothecary shop full of large glass jars with all sort of unidentifiable shriveled and dried things. Signs everywhere were in a beautiful and, to me, indecipherable Chinese script. I wasn't in Kansas. The appointment was unlike any appointment with a Western doctor. Dr. Chao talked to me for less than five minutes, then he had me sit in a chair and he stood behind me and squeezed my head so hard I had to do yoga breathing to keep from yelping. He felt, and pressed hard on, every square millimeter of my scalp and after what seemed like an eternity announced to me that I'd had a traumatic injury to my head when I was an infant and that that was likely the source of my headaches.

What? I couldn't imagine what he was talking about. I'd never had head trauma. I'd never had a brain injury. And then the memories flooded into my brain, the occasional time in my life where my mother had looked at me and said. "You turned out OK. We were worried about you." And I remembered a story in my family about how my father had stumbled at the very top of a set of outdoor concrete stairs to my grandmother's apartment while holding me as an infant, and how I had landed at the bottom of that complete flight of concrete stairs. Well, that explained everything! I felt both horrified, that I'd been suffering from an unacknowledged severe head injury all my life, and relieved, that perhaps this was the answer. He said he thought he could help me. "If I can help you, we'll know after three appointments." Each time he massaged my head very hard. It was excruciating. At first, I thought it did help. But ultimately, the headaches persisted.

My migraines started when I was in the eighth grade. My mother once commented about how she could see I was in pain a block away when I was walking home from school. I didn't know anything about migraines back then. They were bad headaches. I took Tylenol, which didn't really help. I was a good student. I went to school with headaches.

I learned to live with them. I know for certain there are some things that are a headache recipe when I can be one hundred percent sure of getting a migraine, and I avoid those scenarios: Chinese restaurants where the ingredients include MSG—one hundred percent guarantee of a migraine for me. Overindulgence in alcohol—more than two drinks and often even a half glass of wine and I *will* have a migraine in the morning. Any beer, no matter how small the volume, inadequate sleep, being too busy, letting my calendar fill up with too many commitments and obligations. Emotional stress and interpersonal conflict are recipes for migraines, all on their own. And there were always migraines, even when none of these "no-brainer" factors (as I describe them to myself) were in play.

And then, in my fifties, something important happened that seemed at the time completely unrelated.

My friend took me to a party and I met a hypnotist. She told me that people can be helped to stop smoking in as little as one to two sessions. I was amazed. Many people are aware of this fact, I have since learned, but at the time, it was new information for me.

I've been a Registered Nurse for thirty-nine years, most of that time in bedside nursing in Emergency Departments and Intensive Care Units of big hospitals. I've seen a lot of people suffering from end-stage lung cancer, and from the many other ways lungs can fail after years of exposure to smoke. In the final stages, people are bent over with their elbows on their hospital tray-tables, in what we refer to as the "tripod" position: their arms and shoulders supporting their chest, their mind completely focused on the struggle for the next breath. Speaking one word at a time. Hospital rules require me to offer smoking cessation education which always feels to me like a joke because no one ever wants to read it—everyone knows that smoking is bad for you. They just can't stop. We give them nicotine patches, intravenous steroids, and oxygen. My mother died early from lung cancer, having smoked in her younger years. Smoking causes so much suffering. So much loss.

I went home from the party thinking about this new information. Imagine being able to help someone quit smoking in one or two sessions! Could I learn to do that? I spent some time with Google over the next few days, learning that hypnosis was effective for many problems and unwanted behaviors.

Two weeks later, I was standing in Room Two of the Intensive Care Unit where I was employed, taking care of a woman younger than myself detoxing from alcohol. People don't usually die from detoxing from meth or heroin, but they *can* die from alcohol detox, so many patients end up in the ICU where they are monitored every fifteen minutes until they are safely through the dangerous part of detox. My patient was a woman who had once been a beauty queen at the local high school. She'd been drinking hard for many years—she had yellow, jaundiced skin, yellow eyes, and the tell-tale swollen belly of ascites from damage to her liver– so she wouldn't have a normal life span—she was going to die early. And she had alcoholic encephalopathy—even if she did quit drinking, she'd had so much damage to her brain she'd never be able to live independently. I'd taken care of her before—we all had. She was a "frequent flyer," in nursing lingo. She had two daughters, and they'd stopped in for five minutes on their way to high school that morning, kissing her yellow cheek. She was drooling. They acted like nothing was wrong. They had seen her like that so many times. It broke my heart.

As she regained consciousness that day, she got herself out of bed, into her clothes, and tottered unsteadily down the hall and out the door of the hospital, against medical advice. She was headed to the convenience store a block away to get a beer. It wasn't the first time this had happened. I felt frustration flood my body. I really wanted to help her. That's why I became a nurse—to make a difference by helping people. Every time she came in, there was the possibility that this time, she'd dry out, that *this* time she would feel she'd hit "rock bottom," and be ready to change.

It was three-thirty in the afternoon. I remember that because we were short staffed that day and I was hungry. I hadn't taken a lunch break– hadn't wanted to leave her with another nurse who was too busy to watch her carefully. But now she was gone, and I looked around the room at the expensive monitoring equipment, the liter bags of IV fluids and small expensive bags full of drugs on computerized pumps to keep her electrolytes balanced, her vitamin B levels replaced intravenously, her magnesium replaced, sedatives enough to prevent a life-threatening seizure. The trash bin was overflowing with used IV tubing and all the paraphernalia of patient care in the ICU. I couldn't help her. I could prevent her from dying in the ICU over and over, as many times as she wanted to detox, but she wasn't ever going to stop. I felt like a cog in the broken end of the health care system. All this money—taxpayer money—and no-one was benefitting. And at that moment, it was as if a switch flipped in my brain. The experience at the party, the memory of my mother, the intense frustration this day in the Intensive Care Unit... there was another way to help people. I didn't know much about it, but I made a decision at that moment. I decided that I would go anywhere I had to go in the whole world and pay whatever I had to pay to become the best hypnotist I could possibly be, so I could help people *before* their lives and bodies were ruined. I couldn't help that woman—but the world is full of people who need help to quit drinking, to quit smoking—people who could be helped before they got so bad they cycled through the ICU over and over and over, without ever getting better. I could learn to help them quit with hypnosis. I was an experienced nurse, and I knew that what I had been doing as a nurse in a western medicine environment was not working for addictions, or for long term pain management. People were suffering. Now I knew there was a way I could make a difference. I could learn to be a really good hypnotist and make a dent in the suffering, one client at a time.

The next day I applied to Bellingham Technical College, to the yearlong hypnotherapy program. I remembered hearing that there was such a program twenty years ago. I was curious about it back then, but I was nursing full time in the emergency department and had a daughter who was ill. There was no time for exploring hypnosis. The program was still there, still being run by the same teacher, Jami Engholm. She'd been a student of Roy Hunter, who'd been a student of the late Charles Tebbetts. Big names in hypnosis in the United States. I enrolled and I called her on the phone. "You'll never be sorry," she said. "You'll change peoples' lives."

Then I googled hypnosis and hypnotherapy in my community. I wanted to know what it felt like to be hypnotized. What could *I* use hypnosis for? I made an appointment with Erika Flint of Cascade Hypnosis Center, right in Bellingham, where I was living. "What do you want to change about your life?" she asked me. I wanted to sleep better. I wanted to get motivated to finish my three novel drafts. I signed up for a four-session package. I didn't have any idea of what to expect. I just knew I was going somewhere I'd never been and I needed as much experience as possible, from whatever angle I could get it.

Erika had a nice leather recliner in her office for her clients. She put me into a hypnotic trance state by doing a number of different things. She had me push down hard on the arms of the chair and then relax, and then do it again. She picked up my arm and dropped it at one point. She had me repeat some words, quietly and then more quietly. She talked me through a series of relaxation exercises. At one point she told me I couldn't open my eyes, and I tried and I couldn't, so I believed her. And I just remember making a conscious decision to trust her. I wanted to go with her. And then I really relaxed, which was very comfortable, and all I had to do was listen to her voice and follow her instructions. She took me on a sort of guided meditation where there was a fork in the road and we explored what life would be like if I didn't change anything, in one, five, ten years. That was emotionally very uncomfortable. But then we came back to the present day, and she took me up another more challenging but also more fulfilling road where I was sleeping well each night, publishing my first book, where I was playing more harp music, better than ever, and feeling fabulous overall. It just occurred to me as I am writing this that all of these things have come true. I'm not publishing a novel, but I am publishing a book that I hope will help a lot of people, and that's even better. And I notice that even though I am busier than ever—building my hypnosis practice, writing this book—that I have also had more performance opportunities than ever before and I have never played my harp as beautifully as I am playing now.

I left her office that first time feeling clear-headed like my brain had been vacuumed. I saw Erika four times. Each time I left her office I felt elated, with that kind of perspective you get when you go away for the weekend or hike up a mountain and get to look out across valleys and mountains. A kind of big-picture feeling of clarity. I began sleeping better right away.

I wanted to sleep better. I didn't just need to sleep better, I needed to be able to avoid the various nightmare series my brain had been subscribing to all my life. Erika gave me MP3 hypnosis tapes to listen to, to help me relax and to help me go to sleep without the sleep-defying anxious rumination that was my norm.

And almost immediately, I *was* sleeping better, without nightmares. I didn't really know why, then, or *how* all this was happening. I just wanted my life to be better, and it *was* getting better.

I am now a Certified Consulting Hypnotist through the National Guild of Hypnotists, which is the largest and the oldest association of hypnotists in the United States. In the state of Washington, I am registered as a Hypnotherapist. I graduated from the year-long Hypnotherapy program at Bellingham Technical College, which is one of the few formal hypnotherapy programs of that length in the country. Following that foundation, I took the Banyan Hypnotherapy course and became a 5-PATH® Practitioner and a 7th Path Self-Hypnosis® teacher. 5-PATH® and 7th Path Self-Hypnosis® are among the most advanced certifications available. 5-PATH® stands for 5 Phase Advanced Transformational Hypnosis. 7th Path refers to the fact that the Recognitions, or statements which you receive while in hypnosis, may be used 7 different ways. Not long after this, I noticed that as long as I did 7th Path Self-Hypnosis® twice a day, for twenty minutes at a time, I rarely had migraines. The benefits of not having migraine headache pain have changed my life. What could you do with *your* life if you didn't have migraines?

I practice 5-PATH® Hypnosis exclusively because it's an insight-based therapy process that employs advanced hypnosis techniques based on recent developments in brain science. It gets results. Please be aware that my statements about hypnosis are about 5-PATH® Hypnosis and Hypnotherapy. For the purposes of this book, all references to hypnosis are related to the pursuit of health and wellness, so references to hypnosis and hypnotherapy are interchangeable.

I have associate, bachelor's, and master's degrees in nursing, and an MBA. Over the years, I've carried certifications in nursing administration, emergency nursing, and sexual assault examination. I believe in education. Hypnosis is the most interesting topic I have ever studied, and I make it a point to study with experts all over the United States. I spend about a third of my time in scholarly pursuits—attending and speaking at conferences, writing articles for publication, participating in several online study groups, taking courses online and in person. I spend a third of my time seeing clients. I spend a third of my time taking very good care of myself physically, mentally, emotionally, and spiritually, so I can be 100 percent present with my clients. I have a consistent 7th Path Self-Hypnosis® practice which I rely on to keep myself centered and balanced and to keep migraine headaches at bay. I see people for all kinds of problems in my Bellingham office.

"Do you have a view?" my friend asked when she heard I had an office in the tallest building in Whatcom County.

"No, I don't have a view," I said. "I don't have a window. We don't need a view or even windows in the hypnosis office. In the hypnosis office, we look within."

There is a large round mirror in my hypnosis office. We look inside and we see change. It's all about introspection and our subconscious. Self-knowledge, change, releasing old ways of thinking, believing, and being that do not serve us. We gain an understanding of our earlier selves with the wisdom and compassion of our current selves, receiving guidance from our future selves. Forgiving others, forgiving ourselves, setting ourselves free from the emotional chokeholds of past experiences.

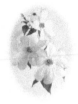

Chapter 3

Overview

My forty-six-year experience of migraine pain has given me a lot of information and understanding. Your experience may be different from mine, but the central core of discomfort and missed opportunities are shared. I managed to escape with hypnosis and self-hypnosis, and I hope you will too. It worked so well for me that now I am committed to helping other people escape the endlessly looping vise grip of migraine headache pain.

In Chapter 4 I'm going to tell you a little about how hypnosis works. Hypnosis is good for lots of problems because lots of problems have at their core some kind of deeply, *subconsciously held* belief or perception that gets the way of enjoying life, and may be expressing itself as pain. Hypnosis works—even when everything else has failed, because it works differently than other approaches to solving your problems—it taps into your powerful subconscious mind where your memories, beliefs, habits, and emotions are. I'll answer the questions you may have. I'll describe what it feels like to be hypnotized.

In Chapter 5 we'll talk about *outside* triggers or things outside ourselves that can cause or contribute to migraine pain. The fact that migraines generally have multiple triggers is new information for some people. You may not realize how many hidden factors are contributing to your migraines. You don't have to identify each and every one to benefit immediately from this knowledge.

Chapter 6 deals with *Inside* triggers. *Inside* triggers include emotions you feel based on thoughts you think—that sounds complicated, but I'll break it down for you. It's a key concept of this book, and one of the primary reasons hypnosis works so well for migraine headache pain. I'll explain how emotional pressure from past experiences, especially from early painful experiences, impacts your life on a daily basis *without you even being consciously aware of it*, and how hypnosis can help you. I'll explain how misperceptions and erroneous responses take up emotional bandwidth in your life that prevents you from living a full and satisfying life, and can contribute to tension and pain. I'll help you identify how limiting beliefs—and we all have them—might be keeping you from enjoying things in your life, and how *this* might actually be contributing to migraine pain.

Chapter 7 is all about the relief of emotional pressure. This is where the magic of 5-PATH® Hypnosis happens. Hypnosis is not magic, but it can feel that way because it works so fast and works so well. What if you don't know the specific causes of emotional pressure? In Chapter 7, we'll go into why these root causes are so difficult to find and resolve using other types of therapies like counseling. I'll share some of the techniques we use to release emotional pressure. We work below the level of your conscious mind, and in a way that your subconscious mind understands and accepts. Your subconscious mind is your memory bank. By following your feelings, your subconscious mind will help you identify the root causes of this emotional pressure. I'll show you how hypnosis can change your perceptions of past events during the hypnosis session, and how this has a positive ripple effect into your present and your future. Changing your beliefs changes your thoughts and behaviors. This is part of the secret of why hypnosis is so fast. Changes are made at a deep level in your mind, and your subconscious mind has the ability to re-adjust the perception of many experiences based on insight from changes made in just a few. This is an example of neuroplasticity, the ability of the brain to learn and change.

I'll explain the value of applying your adult perspective to early events in your life. 5-PATH® Hypnosis is an insight-based process. It is a systematic way of helping you find clarity and wisdom yourself by doing the process with me or with any 5-PATH® Hypnotherapist you trust. The clarity and insight you gain enables change to be instantaneous, and these changes have a ripple effect in your mind, helping you in other areas of your life.

When you know what you should do but can't make yourself do it consistently—hypnosis is good for helping uncover why you have ambivalence, and it helps with motivation. I'll explain misperceptions and erroneous responses to painful events.

I'll explain how limiting beliefs occur, and how they hold you back.

Chapter 8 is about forgiveness, and how important it is to resolve anger. In nearly every spiritual practice, there is an emphasis on the importance of forgiveness. It is widely appreciated. Forgiveness in 5-PATH® has nothing to do with the experience of the offender, and everything to do with *your* experience. Forgiveness is the antidote to anger. Anger carried through a lifetime contributes to all kinds of physical diseases, including depression, when turned inward. Forgiveness allows you to disconnect from the misdeeds of someone in your past. It allows you to go on without carrying anger, hurt, resentment, rage. It frees up tremendous amounts of emotional bandwidth. There is so much more energy to deal with your own life, to do with your life what you want to do. And there is a place for forgiving yourself.

Chapter 9 is about all the ways in which we can get in the way of our own happiness and success in life. It's about using the techniques of hypnosis to uncover ways in which we may be unwittingly perpetuating the cycle of migraine headaches. I'll talk about self-sabotage, and how to know if you are doing it. There may be some side benefits of being unable to participate in your life. You may even be punishing yourself for something. Having headaches might have become a habit so old you don't even remember how it started.

Chapter 10 is about new patterns for a pain-free life and setting yourself up for success. We all have an internal "state" and an internal "soundtrack." Your state is like your emotional temperature gauge—it can be positive or negative, it can be calm and focused with pleasure, or it can be frazzled and panicky. If you are like most people, control of your internal state is not something you learned to regulate well. In fact, most people have not learned to even pay attention to it. It's also the place where your gut feelings or intuition make themselves known. I'll talk at length in Chapter 10 about this. Similarly, the "soundtrack" in your mind, which includes what subject you are focused on and how you are responding to that, and most importantly what you are saying to yourself moment by moment, is very influential in your daily experience. A constant "I'm not good enough/I can't/they won't" thought habit can be damaging beyond belief to your life and, in the worst cases, may have become so habitual you don't even remember ever feeling differently. I'll explain how the "soundtrack" in your mind (what you say to yourself all day long), and the "spin" you put on events around you influences your quality of life every single minute and how important it is for you to consciously make that soundtrack positive.

Being able to identify your internal state and your internal soundtrack is a valuable skill. Being able to change these and manage them is an even more important skill. These skills can make the difference between "just getting through" life and *loving* life, for everyone. And the amazing thing is, neither of these requires different behavior from anyone around you. These are the skills you learn and practice within yourself, which affect your experiences and influence your satisfaction and happiness with your life. And for you, they may have a big impact on the expression of pain in your body.

Chapter 11 is devoted to a De-Stressing Toolkit of seven two-minute stress reduction techniques. If you give these a try, you'll find they are surprisingly easy to learn, and they work! Each one helps you feel better incrementally, and immediately, and each one can be repeated for additional benefit. Some of them are just so simple and give you such a pleasant feeling, you may find you want to do them even when you are not feeling particularly stressed. We live in a fast-paced hectic time, and even a little relief from this intensity is pleasurable. I'll help you figure out ways to make the inclusion of these techniques automatic in your daily life.

Chapter 12 is a discussion of some of the challenges you may face when you are considering using 5-PATH® Hypnosis and 7th Path Self-Hypnosis® to get rid of your migraine headache pain. I'll explain why 5-PATH® Hypnosis is so effective. I'll explain why 7th Path Self-Hypnosis® is so helpful, to cement the changes made in 5-PATH® and to improve your experience of life on a daily basis.

Chapter 13 is a brief summary, intended to help you decide if hypnosis is right for you. There's a lot of information in this book, and at this point, you have quite a bit more information than most of my clients when they begin hypnosis with me. I've included my contact information so that you can reach me if there is anything I can do to give you additional support.

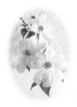

Chapter 4

How Hypnosis Can Work for You

Hypnosis is completely safe. It is a normal and natural state of mind. In fact, you are in and out of a state of hypnosis every day. If you have ever gotten lost in an activity and been surprised to find that so much time has gone by, you have been in the same state of mind that you will be in while we are doing hypnosis together. Any time you lose track of time, you are in a light state of hypnosis. You may have had the experience of driving and missing your freeway exit, or even more disconcerting, suddenly becoming aware that you don't know if you've missed the exit or not—you have no sense of how much time has gone by, or where exactly you are. These are classic examples of "highway hypnosis," when you are actually driving in an altered state of consciousness—a trance state, with eyes gazing at a fixed point. In this state, part of your conscious mind is operating the car and responding to traffic conditions, and another part of your mind is focused elsewhere. This state of mind is very similar to what happens in my hypnosis office, but you will be safely relaxed in a comfortable recliner.

Hypnosis is a state of focused relaxation, and you may have any number of feelings while in hypnosis. You may feel very heavy, or as light as a feather, you may feel very relaxed, or very excited. Some people experience a tingling sensation in their arms and legs. There is not one right way to experience hypnosis—it's different for each person and it can differ from one time to the next.

In hypnosis, you will be alert and conscious the entire time. The only exception to that is if you were using hypnosis to help you through a medical or dental procedure, and then I'd help you be *un*conscious.

Changes made in hypnosis are fast. Our brains learn a phobia quickly, which is just a learned fear, and they can also learn a new way of responding to an old situation. This ability to learn, to change, to heal is called neuroplasticity and is one of the most important new understandings in brain science. It is one of the reasons hypnosis works so well.

Hypnosis is helpful for lots of different problems. In addition to being able to help you experience less pain, it can help you sleep better, and help you break habits of behavior and habits of thought that are detrimental to your happiness. Many people are aware that hypnosis is good for weight loss, and hypnosis is famous for helping people quit smoking. It's helpful for concentration, for passing exams, for public speaking or musical or athletic performance, and for self-confidence. It can help you find lost items and can help you with spiritual growth and to find your purpose in life. It can help you get over a fear of being in elevators or a fear of flying. Hypnosis is a powerful tool that can help you be your best self.

It's helpful, when learning about hypnosis, to understand that there are three parts to your mind. Your conscious mind is your thinking, analytical mind—it's the part of your mind that makes decisions, that compares information, makes judgments, forms opinions. Your subconscious mind is the part of your mind that is your memory bank. It holds all the experiences that have ever happened to you, even though you only remember a fraction with your conscious mind. This is the part of your mind which holds beliefs about yourself and the world around you. This is where your habits reside– both habits of thought and habits of behavior. Your subconscious mind is home to your dreams, imagination, ideas, and emotions. Your emotions are generated by your subconscious mind, in response to your experiences and beliefs. And the third part of your mind is your unconscious. Your unconscious mind is responsible for your heart beating and your blood circulating. It is responsible for your hormone production and keeps all the organs of your body working together harmoniously. It repairs rips in your skin and decides how many white blood cells should be reproduced each day in response to your exposure to germs.

All parts of your mind have protective reflexes to keep you safe and happy. Your unconscious mind has a set of instincts and protective reflexes to keep you safe and secure. It makes you flinch or duck when a ball goes whizzing by your head. Your subconscious mind protects you by habits or by beliefs—sometimes limiting beliefs that serve to protect you from getting hurt, even though they may also be limiting your life. There is also a part of your mind known as the critical factor, a part of your conscious mind, that evaluates new information and decides whether to allow it in, to accept it or not. This is the protective mechanism of your conscious mind, and is the part of your brain that we need to bypass in order to work with your subconscious.

When you watch a film or read a book, you make a conscious decision to "suspend disbelief" in order to be entertained. You consciously decide to bypass the critical factor of your conscious mind.

The primary reason hypnosis is so effective is that it works with your subconscious mind. You may, like most people, believe that your conscious mind is in charge of your life, but you are wrong. It's the other way around. Consider this: you are watching a movie that you've seen before. It features two actors with whom you are familiar. There is a chase scene with high stakes, and you feel your heart racing! Then, there is a scene of interpersonal conflict and you find yourself tense, feeling anxious, and then there is a big loss—someone dies, or the two lovers are separated, with suffering apparent in the faces, voices, and actions of the actors. You notice your eyes are tearing up with emotion. You feel sad. You may even find yourself crying. Now, you *know* that these two actors are actually involved in a child custody dispute and they may be arguing during their break while they are eating fancy sandwiches from a catering truck on the set. You know this. They're just actors. You even know how the movie turns out—everyone is happy. But your heart was *racing*. You were *crying*. Now, isn't that interesting?

So, tell me—what part of you is in control of your body, where you experience your feelings—your conscious mind (actors with everyday lives getting paid big bucks to follow a movie script with a happy ending) or your subconscious mind (something terrible is happening and someone I love is dying). Your sub*conscious* mind is in control. Again, isn't that interesting? You *think* your conscious mind is in control all the time. You are wrong. This is one of the most important things I have to say to you. It explains a lot about how your subconscious mind works and why hypnosis is so fast, and why it is so effective in helping you make changes in your life.

Even if you don't want your subconscious mind to influence your experience of reality, that is what is happening every day, all day. You (like everyone in our society today), believe (and a belief is merely a thought you keep thinking over and over again) and are "thinking" that your conscious mind, your rational, intelligent knowledgeable and experienced mind is in control. Your subconscious mind is the driver for your emotions and your behavior. If our conscious minds were in control of our emotions and behaviors, no one would have any problems changing their behavior, losing weight, or stopping smoking.

If you have struggled with losing weight, then you will identify with this example: You know *exactly* what you should do to lose weight. In fact, you know this so well you could probably write a book about it, because it's simple, right? Eat less, move more. But even though you might want to lose weight more than you want anything else in life right this minute, you are not losing weight. Your conscious, rational mind is not in control. Your subconscious mind is in control. It has a different idea of what will keep you safe and happy, and it leans more toward cheese tortellini than salad.

Before we do hypnosis together, we'll talk about your experience with hypnosis. I'll want to find out what you know about it, and what experience you may have had with it. I will ask you what you most want to work on. Often clients come with several problems, and I always explain that we work on one problem at a time. I will ask you to identify seven benefits to you to make the change you want to make. Seven ways your life will be better, or you will be better. I want you to spend some time thinking about and planning how your life will be different when your problem is no longer part of your life.

You are in control the entire time you are in hypnosis. As your hypnotist, I do not have control over you. Sometimes people say, "Promise you won't make me bark like a dog?" They may be remembering a stage show, perhaps at the county fair, where there was a hypnotist who brought people up on stage and then had them do silly or embarrassing things. This is what I can tell you: I have never felt it was helpful for someone to bark like a dog. And if you want to bark like a dog, you don't need to be hypnotized for that! Think of this: Who would volunteer to be on the stage at a hypnosis show? People who don't mind being the center of attention, who don't mind being on stage when the audience is laughing, who don't mind being videoed by their friends doing something they normally wouldn't do, talked about for weeks afterward. These people are willing to be part of the fun—even if it means they have to do something silly or embarrassing—because it won't be *their* doing—the hypnotist made them do it!

People who come to me for help with something in their life are coming because they want to change. Often they've tried everything. They may have even given up, resigned themselves to the problem they face. And I'm always happy when they've found me because hypnosis works, even when everything else has failed.

Anyone can be hypnotized, as long as you are of normal intelligence and are willing to follow instructions. If you are consciously trying to figure out what is happening and evaluating whether it is working you will miss out on the experience of being hypnotized. Everything has a specific purpose, even though it might seem curious. It is my job as the hypnotist to know whether you are at the right depth for the work that needs to be done. Just follow my instructions. You can go to hypnosis school if you want to know how it works. The important thing is to pay close attention to my voice and follow each and every instruction.

Your experience of being hypnotized will be unique to you, but there are some things that seem to occur for most people. One of the most interesting and surprising things you may notice is that time seems to pass very quickly when you are hypnotized. It is not uncommon at all for me to emerge a client from hypnosis and have them be amazed that an hour or more has passed. It can seem like just a few minutes.

In hypnosis, you might feel very heavy, like you are sinking down into the chair, or you might feel very light, like you could float, like a feather. Sometimes people have a sensation of numbness in their fingertips or toes or a tingling sensation. You might feel the need to cough or to swallow, and this is perfectly fine. You cough and swallow during the night and that does not interrupt your benefit from sleep.

You may need to move in the chair a bit to be comfortable. It is much better to adjust yourself during hypnosis than be distracted by a limb going to sleep or cramping. I generally ask clients if they need to use the bathroom before we start hypnosis. There is something about deeply relaxing that can make you more aware that your bladder is full, and it is distracting to have a full bladder during hypnosis. It is always OK to let me know and I can emerge you so you can visit the bathroom and then re-induce hypnosis when you return. It's not a problem.

You cannot get "stuck" in hypnosis. If there were an emergency situation like a fire alarm during our hypnosis session, you would be able to easily open your eyes and emerge yourself from hypnosis and be able to respond in a normal fashion. And, after hypnosis, you will be able to drive or operate machinery just as if you had not been hypnotized. Hypnosis is perfectly safe. I have a soft warm blanket in my office and encourage you to use it during hypnosis because when you are deeply relaxed you can sometimes feel cold, just as if you were relaxing at home.

So, what's happening in your brain during hypnosis? Your brain has millions of neurons, or brain cells, communicating with each other every second, and that generates electrical activity, or brainwaves, which can be measured in cycles per second, or Hertz (Hz). Brainwaves were first recorded in 1924, and now quite a lot is known about them. There are five basic brainwave patterns and we are all in one of those patterns predominantly all the time. Normal, waking consciousness, when you are alert, reasoning, working, interacting with others, is called the Beta state, and the frequency of Beta waves is 12 to 40 Hz.

Alpha is the next brainwave state, when you are physically and mentally relaxed, daydreaming, not really thinking, at 8 to 12 Hz. If you are lying on the couch half asleep, and you are aware of the dog barking next door or your partner coming in the back door, but you are so relaxed you can't even feel your body, you are in Alpha. In Alpha, you have access to your creativity. Your intuition is available to you in Alpha. Your imagination is heightened. It is the place where you can access deep memories, and where you can experience insight. This is my target for you—deep Alpha and into the edge of Theta.

Theta brainwaves are even slower, 4-7.5 Hz, and this is the state of deep meditation and light sleep. This is where you may experience profound intuition and exceptional insight. Theta is the brainwave state where you may experience a sense of deep spiritual connection or unity with the universe. REM sleep or Rapid Eye Movement sleep occurs somewhere between Theta and Delta and that is when you have active dreaming, whether or not you remember it. Sometimes you may exhibit rapid eye movement during hypnosis. This is perfectly normal and natural.

The fourth brainwave state is the Delta state, a slower brainwave pattern at .5-4Hz. Delta is deep, dreamless sleep. (Interestingly, it is said that yogis who have practiced meditation for a very long time are able to slow their brains to the Delta state and still retain consciousness.) This is the state of sleep where growth and body healing occur.

There is a 5th brainwave state called Gamma—Gamma is an extremely fast (40 Hz) frequency. Gamma waves are what's happening when you are "in the flow," like a musician playing well or an athlete playing well. It's characterized by intense focus with rapid information processing, increased sensory perceptions and memory recall. This is a state of peak performance. Gamma waves are present even during REM sleep and sometimes during visualization. Although we are in one of these patterns primarily all the time, there may be other wave states mixed in.

Hypnosis is safe and comfortable. You are in a state of hypnosis quite naturally every evening on your way to sleep. When you get ready for bed, you are probably in Beta, as you arrange your belongings for the morning, brush your teeth, set your alarm. As you read your book for a few minutes, you are in low Beta, and as you turn out your light, you descend from low Beta to Alpha, to Theta, and finally to Delta. It is a very pleasant feeling to feel your consciousness descending—that delicious feeling of falling asleep when you are very tired. And going into a hypnotic trance—and trance is just an older word for brainwave state—a synonym is *daydream*– is generally a very pleasant sensation.

I start out all hypnosis sessions by asking your permission to hypnotize you. I ask if I may touch your finger, hand, arm, possibly forehead. During hypnosis, there may be times when I suggest you communicate with me by moving your finger. At times during hypnosis, I may be looking for a yes or no answer and when you are deeply hypnotized, speaking can sometimes feel like too much work, and moving your finger seems easier than talking. I may pick up your arm and drop it. This is a classic deepening technique developed by Dave Elman. It seems rather mysterious that just having your arm lifted and dropped helps you go more deeply relaxed, but it works. And it is a very pleasant sensation. I may rock your head from side to side. Head rocking is another pleasant sensation that can help you become more deeply relaxed. I may tap on your forehead to help you focus from time to time. I may press down on your shoulder, or touch your hand. I will let you know ahead of time when I do these things so I don't startle you. There are specific reasons for these things, and again, you can always go to hypnosis school if this is the most interesting part of this discussion for you. Meanwhile, just follow the instructions carefully. The important thing is that the induction is designed to assist you into a brain wave state where you can accept helpful suggestions and where you have access to subconscious information so that you can solve the problems you came to the hypnosis office to solve. I know how to tell what level of hypnosis you are in and exactly what to do to adjust this, so you have access to your subconscious mind and the most insight. Clients always feel good when they emerge from hypnosis. It feels good letting yourself sink into a deeper brainwave state and when you emerge, you've just had a nice, refreshing rest. And having the experience of insight during hypnosis—of small bits of wisdom, simple truths—or discovering some new understanding about yourself can leave you feeling exhilarated.

Right now, as you are reading this, or as I am talking with you prior to hypnosis in my office, you and I are in Beta. It is my job to guide you into Alpha, and into the edge of Theta, deep enough to have bypassed the critical factor and deep enough for you to access your subconscious memories and gain insight. In hypnosis, you can become aware of things you are not aware of in your normal waking consciousness. It is your job to listen carefully to my voice, to follow directions, and to relax as much as possible.

The starting place for doing hypnosis is the induction. The induction is a series of exercises that help you become deeply relaxed. As you become deeply relaxed physically, you can become deeply relaxed mentally. Hypnotists sometime use the word sleep, and by that, we mean to go deeply relaxed as if you were asleep. If you close your eyes and reach for that feeling of sleep, and listen closely to the voice of your hypnotist, you are halfway there.

The induction process is, in a way, brain entrainment. The most beautiful and classic example of brain entrainment is a lullaby. The mother sings her awake children to sleep by starting with a melody at a pace that keeps their interest, and by capturing their attention with a story. She proceeds to sing more slowly and more softly. She is *entraining* their brains, leading them to a place of slower brainwaves, specifically from Beta to Alpha and to Theta and on to Delta. She doesn't know those details. The important thing is, it works. And when you see me or any other hypnotist you trust, you do not need to understand the mechanics to make good use of the results.

Hypnotists make use of the concept of brain entrainment. I use my voice, the volume, the pitch, and the cadence, to help you transition from a Beta state of waking consciousness to the relaxed Alpha state, and then to the edge of Theta. And it can feel like being sung to. After several times in my chair, you may have the sense of a familiar bedtime story, and it helps you relax more deeply, and faster. I like my clients to listen to my relaxation MP3 ahead of hypnosis because they become familiar with my voice and associate my voice with relaxation. The brain entrainment begins before I even see some clients for their first session. This is very beneficial for clients. There are a lot of different inductions, a lot of different ways to do this. I learned some of the most sophisticated and effective inductions in existence which are based in time-tested hypnosis history and also in modern neuroscience. In your first session with me, I will be determining which induction techniques work most comfortably and effectively for you. It's your job to relax, to follow instructions, which is mostly listening to what I say and thinking about the things I suggest to you. You will hear every word I say. Even if you get very, very relaxed and start to fall asleep, I will know this and I will pull you back so that you get the benefit of everything you came to me for.

The most important concept about 5-PATH® is that it is an insight-based process. I assist you in finding basic truths—little bits of wisdom—about yourself and your life. I am a guide of sorts, into your subconscious mind. I will guide you into an Alpha brainwave state where everything that has happened to you is available to you. This is the realm of your mind where you have access to understanding, to know the origins of fears, beliefs, behaviors, thoughts. It's all available to you. We have to bypass your conscious mind, sometimes referred to as your monkey mind, your rational mind, the part of you that is constantly judging whether something is true or not, whether you should believe it and accept it or not. So in hypnosis, we duck below this level and communicate at the subconscious level.

We don't say "wake up" from hypnosis because hypnosis is not sleep. I will emerge you from hypnosis, slowly, usually with a leisurely count from one to five. I will guide you. You don't have to wonder how you'll know when it's over. I will be crystal clear. You will probably be very surprised to notice how much time has gone by. Many of my clients, especially the first time, report that the session felt like twenty minutes when in fact they were hypnotized for over an hour!

Most people feel a slight sense of euphoria upon emerging from hypnosis. The inner knowing that you bring back with you from a hypnosis session is valuable and special, and it feels good. It is very satisfying to feel progress is being made on an important issue in your life. It is gratifying to know that a problem you may have struggled with for years is being resolved. You feel confident that you can change your experience of life, and have a better, happier, and more pleasurable life. Connecting the insights from 5-PATH® hypnosis to your migraine headaches can be life-changing.

In the case of migraines, the pain is caused by vasodilation—an expanding of microscopic blood vessels in your brain. This is occurring at an *un*conscious level. But as we saw in the movie example, your body responds to your *thoughts*. What is happening in your mind—in your "state" of mind, and your internal "soundtrack," or what you are saying to yourself inside your head is played out in your body. This is not a new idea—everyone knows that unmanaged stress can express itself in all sorts of ways in our bodies— famously in cardiovascular disease and heart attacks. And there is research to prove that ICU patients heal faster in an environment where the doctors and nurses are getting along. How you *feel* and what you *say* to yourself has an enormous impact on your health, and for *you*, on your *headaches*.

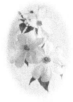

Chapter 5

Outside Triggers

There are multiple triggers contributing to migraine pain, and everyone's experience is different. In this chapter, I'll remind you of some of the common triggers which might be easy for you to avoid. I'm also considering triggers from your own body, like hormonal changes, to be external triggers because you are going to use external strategies to deal with them. Then in the next chapter, we'll dive into internal triggers, to things happening inside your mind, in both your conscious and subconscious minds that can be addressed using hypnosis.

Just like there are many triggers that contribute to migraine pain, there are many different things you can do to help prevent migraines. I suggest you "cast a wide net," using all the support available to you. Start with your doctor, to rule out other problems that could be causing pain in your head. Find out if you have other health problems that need attention. Find out if you have hormone imbalances or fluctuations that could be contributing to tension and migraines. It is stressful to your body to have any kind of illness. If you have access to a formal pain clinic, take advantage of this. You may already have some ideas of what triggers you. You may know what things make it likely that you will get a headache, just based on your own experience, and this is very valuable information and an excellent place to start. It's not important to understand every last thing that can cause or contribute to a migraine.

There are easy to implement strategies to reduce the likelihood of a migraine. You already know some of these. Muscle tension: many people carry tension in their bodies, experiencing a sore neck, or a sore back. Physical tension can be relieved to a degree by moderate exercise. Patients in hospitals can get sore and stiff just from being relatively immobile in bed, and often can get relief from a few trips around the nurses' station.

Our bodies are designed for physical movement, yet many of us have lifestyles that don't allow for regular use of all our muscles. Enlisting the help of a gym or an organized group like a biking or hiking or walking group can be helpful in managing this. You can get guidance from a teacher in a yoga or stretching or tai chi class, or any kind of exercise class that fits your interests and abilities. There are lots of people who make their living helping people be more comfortable in their bodies. Bodywork therapies like chiropractic care, acupuncture, massage therapy, and craniosacral therapy are a few things that can help. And there are healthy ways to help yourself get more movement and flexibility into your life that do not have any cost associated with them—talking a walk after dinner or first thing in the morning, or anytime. The point is, your body needs to move, and movement and stretching can help dissipate tension. We live in a society where people, as a rule, do not get enough exercise. Some people feel that time is a constraint in their attempt to get movement and exercise into their lives, but you can fit small amounts of anything into your schedule. Moving your body is key.

Some people experience triggers related to air temperature, or air quality, suffering if they are exposed to second-hand smoke or summer heat. Make arrangements in your life so you can be prepared to make adjustments as needed.

Being inadequately nourished is also stressful to your body. Poor nutrition and dehydration are well known environmental triggers. Get the junk food and food preservatives out of your diet. And transition to an organic diet—at least for the dirty dozen. I put myself on a vegan, dairy free diet for six months just to see what it was like, and I noticed almost immediately that despite changing 100 percent to more expensive organic produce, my grocery bill decreased noticeably. The meats and dairy products were expensive. I felt very comfortable on a vegan, dairy free diet. I had plenty of energy, and I wasn't hungry all the time like I half expected to be. I lost a few pounds without effort. Cut back on your meat and dairy and put the savings toward 100 percent organic produce.

In a country where safe water is available everywhere, it is surprising to realize that lots of people are dehydrated. I noticed from fifteen years' experience in emergency departments that everyone feels better after receiving a liter of intravenous fluid. We live in a hectic time, and we sometimes forget to put our needs first. Water is essential for life. We all know this. Drink real water. Get the chemicals out of your beverages. There are some things that are so harmful, even if not specifically being a trigger, that I recommend you eliminate them from your diet. Diet sodas are an excellent example. It is not necessary for you to have a degree in chemistry to understand health concerns about how artificial sweeteners break down into formaldehyde, and how these substances affect gut bacteria and glucose intolerance. The real takeaway is this simple truth: your body needs water, every day. *Clean* water in adequate amounts. If you feel thirsty, you are already dehydrated. You need water, not diet soda, not energy drinks. I call these the "no-brainers."

There are a lot of daily habits that are easy to change just by focusing our awareness on them and reminding ourselves of how important they are. Just making the decision to change is powerful. Many habit-improving changes are relatively easy to make (others require hypnosis).

Sleep! Sleep is so important. Sleep "hygiene" is as important as physical hygiene. We all learned to brush our teeth every day, to prevent cavities. Most of us learned to go to bed at a reasonable hour early in life, to get adequate rest, but we don't always do that now. Here is a condensed sleep protocol:

- Eat your last meal early enough that you are not busy digesting food when you lay down to sleep. It's a good idea to give your body a break from active digestion for at least twelve hours every night. Give it a rest!
- Avoid caffeine after noon if it keeps you awake at night.
- Cut back on or avoid alcohol.
- Cut back on sugar.
- Avoid hectic or stressful activities at the end of the day.
- No screens phones/tablets/computers/TV for the last two hours of your day.
- Keep the lights low.
- If you are worried about your to-do list for the next day, it can be helpful to write it down and get it out

of your brain. It will be there in the morning, and you will be refreshed and ready for it.

- Quiet music for relaxation or meditation recordings are readily available on the internet.
- Your hypnotherapist may have a recording to help you sleep.
- Keep the temperature of your sleeping area comfortable.
- Choose your bedtime so you have enough time to get adequate rest before your alarm goes off in the morning.
- Enlist the help of people in your household. Ask for what you want. You deserve to get good rest each night.

Disconnect from unpleasant sources of stress. You don't have to be at the mercy of every stimulus around you. When I started my hypnosis education, I was still working full time as an ICU RN. I knew I was in for a particularly busy year. I decided to take a news holiday for a year. At the time it seemed like all the news was negative, some of it was actually scary, and every news bulletin was a variation on an unpleasant and disappointing theme. I have friends who check the news several times a day. I knew if anything happened that needed my personal attention, they would let me know. Of course, I would come out of my retreat if I needed to inform myself adequately to participate in an election, but it did not help the world and it certainly did not help me to be aware of political changes hour by hour. At the end of the year, the political scene was pretty much the same, but I was relaxed, having put my attention and time into projects that were helping me develop and grow and enjoy life. Some people around me had been tied up in knots for the past year, complaining about how stressed they were. There are people in our society who are very good at working on improving the political climate. I'm not one of them. We only have control over one thing—where we put our attention and how we choose to respond to what we perceive. *You* make the choice for yourself. Don't let people and situations around you make that choice.

Make it a point to look for positive things all around you, in other people, in situations. This is a key to having sovereignty over your "state"– to having control over how you feel instead of being at the mercy of everything you hear and everything you see.

Change the mental channel in your head when you go home. Make your home as comfortable and welcoming as you can. Your home is your nest. Make it beautiful. Get yourself organized so you can find your belongings easily. Marie Kondo wrote a charming book entitled *The Life Saving Magic of Tidying Up*. She talks about only having things in your home that spark joy.

Enjoy the beauty of the earth. The Japanese culture has a lovely tradition of "Forest Bathing"—just a walk in the forest, in the quiet peacefulness, listening to birds and tree branches moving, feeling the texture of the trail or road under your feet can be soothing and relaxing, kind of like hitting the "reset" button.

Give yourself a "time out." In some families and schools, children are given a "time out" to help them regain their composure. That sounds delicious to me. A quiet twenty-minute nap on my desk after lunch sounds good. Give that to yourself. Set your phone timer for twenty minutes and just sit with your eyes closed and imagine your body on a warm beach, the sun and air temperature perfect, and just let yourself sink down. Or just enjoy the pleasure of your own bed or couch, throw a blanket over yourself and just have a twenty-minute rest, sinking into the comfort of your own private haven from the busy world. In the back of this book is a link to a twenty-minute hypnosis MP3 I recorded, which you may download. It's the equivalent of a nap. If you listen to it, (use stereo headphones to get full advantage of the binaural beats) you will feel rejuvenated.

You can also give yourself permission for an emotional holiday "just for today." Let people and situations that normally bother you roll off your back, just like water beading up and rolling off the back feathers of a duck. Nothing can get under your skin and bother you. Just decide to give yourself a break. Give yourself permission to take a holiday from trying to help other people in your life. You don't have to get the whole thing right, forever. Just for today.

You may already know there are changes you need to make in your life around the work you do or the people you spend time with. I love Mary Oliver's question, *"Tell me, what are you going to do with your one wild and precious life?"* As far as we know, we get just one life on earth. If the work you do, if the way you spend your hours, if the people you spend your hours with are not fulfilling to you, then you need to focus on making changes. If this is the case, just reading this will resonate with you. Listen to yourself. Big changes start with *the next smallest thing*. What can you do to start some forward momentum, to start making important changes in your life?

Solitude Days. One of the best gifts I give myself is a Solitude Day. I try to do this once a month. I spend twenty-four hours at home, alone, without talking to anyone, without getting into my car. It's usually a pajama day. No phone, no computer, no internet, no phone calls, no texting. I avoid electronics. I try to avoid electricity (I do make an exception for my coffeepot in the morning…this is supposed to be a pleasurable exercise, after all!).

Your first time it might be slightly uncomfortable—just the thought of not having your phone, friends, and the world readily available. Give it a try. I purposefully do not have a to-do list for this day. No chores. The only thing on my list is my relaxation and pleasure. I often spend some time outside in nature, sitting and enjoying my garden. I might do some light gardening in the warm months if I feel like it, sometimes just cutting flowers and making a particularly nice bouquet. I might fill the bird feeders with seeds and replace suet blocks. This is a wonderful time to give yourself permission to play with your art supplies. Just doodling around is fun, making a mess and not worrying about Getting Things Done. I light candles at dusk and spend my evening by candlelight. Candlelight slows you down. When you can't see past the candlelight, you can't be reminded of all the things that need doing in your house. It's less stimulating to your conscious mind. It's relaxing to your subconscious mind. I read, or write in my journal. I might give myself a pedicure. Only if I feel like it. I go to bed early and enjoy the added benefit of a very good night's rest.

Life is busy. You'll likely have to schedule this in advance. If you have children, make arrangements for their care with a friend or relative. Those adults might be inspired to try their own Solitude Day after seeing how you benefitted. If you have other adults living with you, try to arrange to be alone as much as possible. If someone else sleeps at your house and you can't make arrangements otherwise, sleep in a different room and ask them to observe silence and take a break from eye contact. The first week-long writing retreat I ever attended included a thirty-six-hour period of silence, and I noticed the more experienced retreat attendees did not even have eye contact with each other at meals. They were respectfully choosing not to intrude into other people's creative process. You need solitude. Alternatively, you could go away and rent a cabin on a beach. Once I went camping on the stormy Washington coast in October, alone. I had the beautiful windswept beach to myself for two days. But my favorite place is the comfort of home.

I often make a garden mandala to ceremonially mark time as my own. This is easy and I am always surprised by how much I enjoy it. It takes about twenty minutes: You'll need a container—a basket is nice, or a bowl or even a paper grocery bag. Take a pair of scissors and go outside. Look for shapes and colors. Collect leaves, pine cones, long blades of grass, flowers, petals, seed pods, buds, anything beautiful you find. Then go back inside and arrange the items in a concentric circle. I often start with a circle about six inches in diameter using one of the botanical bits I have brought in, maybe small yellow birch leaves. Then segments of red stem from a bush outside my back door. Then I decorate the tip of each stem with a small pinecone. I might then make a circle of lavender stems all the way around. Whatever you brought in, you can use. Just put the different colors and shapes in a pattern that pleases you. The simple act of making concentric circles of one color after another is easy and very pleasing. Don't think it through—don't plan it. Just keep your hand moving, enjoying all the shapes and hues. Lay everything down in circles, one after the other. If you are inspired to make the pattern more complex, do it—as long as it feels fun and playful. You are engaging your right hemisphere. This helps you get out of your conscious mind and into your subconscious mind, where you are in a position to feel relaxed and dreamy, creative, and insightful. You can use all the flowers, but you don't need to. You don't need to make a dent in your garden or your neighbor's garden. There are beautiful bits of nature that blow off trees. The petals of a rose nearly spent is a source of a beautiful ring of soft color. I like to create these mandalas by my door— either outside or in. I think of it as my "Beauty Gate." No one can get to me without going through the Beauty Gate, and I have to give my permission. I am safe and secure in my cocoon for the day.

It is very important for you to give yourself sources of pleasure and enjoyment. Pleasure and enjoyment help your body and your mind relax. Try new things. Take a yoga class, take a walk in a new place. Start a relaxing hobby or a fun activity you've been putting off. Many people deny themselves pleasurable activities. Even if you are very busy with a lot of responsibilities, you can find thirty minutes once a week for your own project. There are so many ideas, the most difficult part might be choosing just one to start with.

Practice saying no to other people so you can say YES! to yourself. You hear this all the time, and we all "get" this concept, but lots of us have a hard time doing it. I love this quote from Anne Lamont: "Oh, my G*d, what if you woke up one day and you're sixty-five or seventy-five, and you never got your memoir or novel written, or you didn't go swimming in warm pools and oceans all those years because your thighs were jiggly and you had a nice comfortable tummy or you were just so strung out on perfectionism and people-pleasing that you forgot to have a big juicy life? Don't let this happen."

Not knowing what you should do differently is an education opportunity for yourself. Learn how to get enough sleep. Learn about healthy food.

Knowing what you should and want to do differently, but not doing it—like *I know I should go to bed earlier but I keep staying up*– or *I know I shouldn't work so many extra hours but I keep doing* it is an opportunity for hypnosis to help you. There are likely subconscious reasons why you are not doing something you know you should be doing, or doing some things you know you should not be doing.

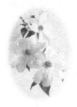

Chapter 6

Inside Triggers

This is where hypnosis will help you the most. Hypnosis can help you stay on your plan to manage all the external triggers, but the real value is identifying internal triggers and eliminating those triggers using hypnosis and the power of your subconscious mind. Internal conflicts consume a lot of energy and there is great value in subconscious resolution.

Pain is an important way your body communicates with you. And on some level, there is a deep knowledge that if there is pain, there must be something wrong. And if there is *severe* pain, as with migraine headache pain, then some part of us will naturally be fearful that there is something *severely* wrong. Please remember, as I mentioned in my introduction, I require that your doctor give permission before I will work with you to take away your pain. Once your doctor is satisfied that there is nothing more seriously wrong, and nothing more he or she can do to help you eliminate migraine headache pain, then I can safely and ethically work with you to help you manage and hopefully eliminate your headache pain.

You may be paralyzed by the fear of pain—I know I was, at times. I found myself feeling hopeless. Fear of pain influences your physical experience of pain. Your history of pain influences your current experience with pain. Mistaken beliefs about pain influence the current experience. You have laid down a neural pathway where thoughts and feelings lead to migraine pain. You've done this for so long, the pathway has become a rut in your brain. Ruts are hard to get out of. And the process of following those pathways over and over again has become so automatic that you don't even realize you are doing it.

I'll encourage you to remember that pain is temporary in most cases. I know how hard this is to believe in the midst of a headache, but it is. It's temporary. And although some pain may be inevitable, the suffering is optional. And I'll help you learn how to use the role of your attention in managing your discomfort. Managing your *state* and managing your *soundtrack* is key. And I will give you some specific tools to help you set yourself up for the success of less pain.

Changing your perceptions, which are the conclusions you reached based on what you saw, felt, or experienced, changes your beliefs. And beliefs are just thoughts you think over and over again.

Mistaken perceptions can color your entire life, making things harder than they need to be. I want to share an example of this from my own experience when I first learned 7th Path Self-Hypnosis®. We were all laying on the floor of the classroom, with the lights off. We were going back, under hypnosis, to a very early time when we felt loved. Going back to that time and feeling, reaching for the felt memory of actually being there. I immediately found myself on my fourth birthday receiving a gift from my paternal grandmother, Meggie. I remember reaching up to her as she leaned down, handing me a card with sparkly glitter. How did she know I loved glitter? Then she handed me the most beautiful doll I had ever seen in my life. I felt so loved, so understood. She knew just exactly what I liked! I looked down at my feet and saw my bare four-year-old feet on the wood floor. Then I looked over my shoulder, to my room down a short hallway. I saw the doorknob to my bedroom and it was just above my eye level! At that moment, I realized that, in my adult brain, I was seeing this from the perception of my four-year-old self. Right behind this flash of surprise, I felt the forgotten memory of what had happened right after I received the doll. I remembered wanting more than anything in the world to go home with Meggie and live with her. She was so smiling and calm and she understood me. This was in sharp contrast to my experience with my mother. My mother was tense and angry. I asked if I could live with Meggie. My mother was *so* angry. I learned that would *not* be an option. And behind this unearthed memory came a flash of insight. That's why I became an overachieving perfectionist. After that experience, I decided to be a good girl, to please my mother, and that is how this need expressed itself in my life. There are worse things. That drive to be perfect led to a successful career. Perfectionism is a good quality in an Intensive Care Unit Nurse. It's a good quality in a nursing administrator with a million details to keep track of, a multimillion-dollar budget, and more than a hundred employees. But I never understood why I am the way I am. In that split second, I had complete self-knowledge. I emerged from hypnosis in tears, but I felt grateful for the insight. I had always carried a conscious memory of the pleasure of receiving the sparkly card and the beautiful doll, but the rest of the experience had been buried in my subconscious. I experienced a more complete version of this deep memory and the emotional experience that went with it. Because this was, in fact, an age regression, I had the viewpoint of my adult self at the same time I re-experienced the event from the perspective of my four-year-old self. From that, I experienced a flash of insight, of self-knowledge. I had, while lying on the floor in the classroom, the adult perspective of that moment. I had the adult future knowledge that the four-year-old me did not know or understand.

I turned four on December twenty-seventh, two days after Christmas. Holidays can be stressful in any household. My sister had been born eight days earlier. My mother and her mother-in-law Meggie had never been on friendly terms. My innocent request to live with Meggie was fuel on an already burning fire. But my mother's outraged response had such an impact on me that it led to a personality expression I might not otherwise have had. And this experience demonstrates how I internalized a volatile experience at the age of four that set me down a life path. Now I know that my mother's angry reaction had very little to do with me, and much more to do with her conflict with her mother in law, and the fact that she was eight days postpartum with a second child in the middle of a major holiday. She was only twenty-five years old. Now I have such compassion for all of us. Self-knowledge is so valuable.

I have since felt more compassion for myself, for how hard I tried to be a successful child in my mother's household. I understand how I came to be the way I am. This mistaken perception, that I had to be perfect to have my mother's approval, shaped my life. She would have been dismayed to learn how this early experience shaped my understanding of how the world worked and my understanding of my place in the world.

Unfortunately, there are many opportunities in life for children to step away from an experience with a mistaken perception. Some children step away with fear or anger or shame or guilt. The important takeaway is that, looking at those situations with our adult perspective, none of us would agree that the child in the situation should be carrying the heavy loads. Those loads belong to the adults in the situation. But I have seen over and over with my clients that they have picked up heavy loads that were not theirs to pick up. And they suffered for years as result. Our adult selves now would know that the conclusion we drew from our childhood experience was flawed, but we didn't have our adult perspective when we were children. These *mistaken perceptions* can change the course of your life. Mistaken perceptions may have made you feel responsible for things no child should ever feel responsible for. You didn't have the understanding or even the vocabulary to express this when you were young. You may not have conscious awareness of the details of the event and how they made you feel in the moment, and how they impacted you. My experience with the doll and my mother's reaction to my request is a good example. There isn't a way to get at these from your conscious mind. Hypnosis is such a valuable tool.

Changing your perceptions changes your beliefs. Changing your beliefs changes how you experience events, and how you experience relationships. Changing how you experience events and relationships changes your behavior, your habits. How you experience events—how you assign *meaning* to events—changes your internal soundtrack, what you say to yourself all day. It changes your thought habits, as well as your behavior habits.

In the next chapter, I'll tell you more about how you can change your perceptions of things that are happening to you now, and things that have happened to you in the past. In the example above, the age regression experience gave me a deep understanding of how difficult that day was for my mother, and how the seed was planted that day for part of my personality. I feel more relaxed now about my conscious memories of tumultuous days in my childhood. I consciously as well as subconsciously have extrapolated that memory and experience to many other situations in my early childhood when she was angry with me. This is a subtle, but important change. There was nothing wrong with me. I was adorable like all little children are adorable.

Chapter 7

Relief of Emotional Pressure

There is tremendous value in applying your own wisdom to events from your past. In a simplistic example, imagine you have a small child who awakes screaming from her "experience" of monsters under her bed. You gather her up, giving physical and emotional reassurance, you turn on the light, you get down and look under the bed, you change the story of her experience "those monsters aren't really there—you are safe—we'll leave this night light on and monsters cannot come near when there is a night light or a stuffed animal that is a protector. You tell her a story that her child mind will accept. Now she goes back to sleep. Now she knows she has a tool, a nightlight, a brown stuffed horse, and the support of her parent if the monster tries to fool her again.

Another child may have this same experience of monsters, but lay alone and awake, terrified, and have sleeping problems throughout life as an adult, perhaps unaware of the memory of under-bed monsters or at least not connecting the pervasive anxiousness in her life with that one event.

Consider this: If you had a young person in your life that you loved dearly, would you want them to have had this experience? Wouldn't you want them to understand that they were lovable, that there was nothing wrong with them, and that 100 percent of the responsibility for whatever difficult experience happened in their early life is the grownup's responsibility? What do you wish you had known then that you know now? And what does that young version of yourself need to know to survive this emotionally? It would be helpful if they knew they were cared for, loved, noticed, appreciated, that there was someone, even if only the older version of themselves, who had deep compassion for them. Feeling completely alone is horrible, and it can be devastating for a small child.

Having a problematic habit of thought or behavior does not mean that something terrible happened to you as a child. Not every habit of thought or behavior is based on an early traumatic event, as we would characterize it as adults today. Some of my clients have found the earliest memory of emotional distress may be something as seemingly benign as hearing their parents fighting repeatedly in the next room. As grownups, we know while this is unpleasant, it's not a life-threatening experience. But to a pre-verbal child, this experience can feel absolutely life-threatening and can be the worst experience of their life up until that point.

Something which seems as simple and commonplace as waking up alone in the dark and screaming and not having someone come immediately to comfort them can also seem life-threatening and can stimulate perfectly natural self-soothing behaviors. Some of these continue, sometimes changing in details, into adult life, manifesting as habits of behavior: skin picking, nail-biting, thumb sucking. Some of these become habits of thought, like a pervasive lack of self-confidence or a feeling that "I don't matter" or "I'm not good enough (to warrant attention, comforting, a feeling of safety)." But going back to a deep memory, and taking your adult self with you can lead to insight which is powerful and life-changing.

Hypnosis can provide you with the opportunity, at a subconscious level, to connect with yourself and provide support for that younger version of you. In hypnosis, your adult self can talk with your child self or even your infant version of yourself, providing listening, acceptance, understanding, information, and perspective. That experienced connection of trust, of love, of compassion, is extremely powerful in defusing the internal tension you may have been carrying, possibly for decades.

Some people feel fearful that hypnosis might uncover past experiences that are too painful and might stir up uncomfortable feelings. There are a number of ways a skilled hypnotherapist will handle this. There is research to show that when you take an experience out of context and review it, adding information to it from the viewpoint of your adult self, it changes the memory of that experience. There are hypnosis techniques to help you with this, techniques to anchor you in the hypnosis chair. If something difficult happened to you as a child, viewing that event remotely, as if seeing it play out on a small black and white screen, can give you access to the memory without reactivating the emotions. You still have the opportunity to inform your younger self that you are going to get through this experience, that you are loved, by your older self even if by no one else, and you can tell your younger self whatever you need to tell her to help her get through the situation and feel loved and supported. If nothing else, you will tell her that one day she'll be grown up and a lot of good things are going to happen along the way. You will tell her that she will grow up with compassion for other people who have difficult experiences. This conversation with her future self changes her experience and has a ripple effect in her brain—in your brain.

In the simplest terms, you are going back in time, under a hypnotic trance that lets you access all the memory and insight of your subconscious mind. You are taking with you your adult self, your adult experience, your adult perspective, and your adult intention of supporting and comforting your younger self, and you are giving your younger self support, encouragement, and helpful advice. At the same time, you are receiving this support, encouragement, and helpful advice from the perspective of your younger self, from your older self. You have this experience from both perspectives at once. The first part of what we do in the hypnosis office helps you understand the details around these earlier events.

In the case of Janey, she was able to take back to her toddler self the adult knowledge that her parents were so different they probably should never have even been married, and that her father had an anxiety disorder and that her mother was young and unprepared and unsupported in her own life for the responsibilities of motherhood. There was absolutely no intention by either of them to hurt Janey. Both her parents wanted the best for her, yet toddler Janey had felt like she might die at any minute. She also felt like she was never able to be good enough—because if she was "good" enough, then her parents wouldn't be fighting all the time. You can see the twisted logic with which a toddler might interpret the world around her. Her emotional response led to behaviors which continued throughout her life. They became habits which persisted into her adult life, inexplicable, and seemingly from nowhere. When adult Janey felt threatened, stressed, or uncomfortable in any way, she bit her nails. Somehow the nail-biting felt somewhat comforting. Her brain was looking for comfort. The scary feeling occurred, she bit her nails and felt momentary comfort. This nail-biting did not *solve* the problem. It provided a *distraction* from the feeling, but in doing that, it also provided some small measure of relief. To the brain, looking always for economy—for the fastest solution to any problem—the fact that this behavior worked, even if only for a moment, wired that connection in her brain. Over time, this became a pathway in her brain that was so frequently traveled that it became a rut– hard to get out of. Any discomfort, and nail-biting, or the urge to bite nails, followed.

Your brain—all parts of your brain—your conscious mind, your subconscious mind, your unconscious mind— all like to do the least amount of work possible to achieve the outcome desired. In nature, the path of least resistance is a recurring theme. A river flows downhill, moving gently around objects that get in its way. An animal will not chase a prey target when the anticipated effort is greater than the caloric reward. Your mind operates similarly. If you feel bad about something and you can distract yourself with "too much" of anything—food, smoking, drinking, text/screen time, working too much, shopping too much, gambling too much, then you temporarily have successfully escaped the bad or uncomfortable feeling. That was a successful strategy, in terms of your brain. Your brain is likely to want to do it again next time you feel bad. Because you *do* feel good, for the moment. Your brain gets the feedback that yes, the cookie /the beer/ the cigarette/the extra time on Facebook/ extra hours at work/twenty dollars in the slot machine/etc. all *do* make you feel better in the short run. Now, these events did not really solve the problem of the moment. They were merely distractors. But you *do* feel better for a moment. Your brain's assessment is *mission accomplished!* Now your *conscious* mind might not agree if you gain twenty pounds, become an alcoholic, smoke a pack a day, spend so much time on your screens that you miss out on real-life pleasures, work so much your family complains, shop or gamble too much, wasting time and money. And this doesn't really have to happen very many times to set up a repetitive pattern. Your brain is clever and learns fast. This is the feel bad-distract cycle that Cal Banyan describes in *The Secret Language of Feelings*. The problem is that every time these things are paired—for one person it is feel bad, eat a cookie; for another, it is feel bad, have a drink—every time those two events are paired, that relationship is strengthened. In neuroscience, they say, "what fires together wires together." So after a while, it's just automatic for you to eat a cookie or have a drink. You have paved a pathway through the neurons of your brain. After months and years of this, it is almost impossible to do anything else. This is why habits have control over you, and why they are so seemingly impossible to change.

In hypnosis, we have to accomplish two important tasks at the same time to break that strong bond of bad feeling–

unwanted behavior. First, we use your powerful subconscious mind to find the root of the uncomfortable or bad feeling, and we deal with it at a subconscious level. And second, we put up a neurological roadblock and chart a new path through your brain.

Back to the smoking example. You feel slighted, bored, or unappreciated (or after a while, *any* uncomfortable feeling can get included in the triggers that lead to a cigarette), and you find yourself smoking. We'll reach back into your life and revisit the origin of you starting to smoke. We can even use the power of your imagination to have a conversation with that long-ago version of you. We can give that younger version of yourself information that you probably wish now you'd know back then. We could be sure that version of you knows how unhappy this habit is making you now. We would probably have some helpful advice to help you through whatever life experience you were distracting yourself from, too. And you are likely to believe this advice, trust it, and accept it, because it is actually coming from you, someone who knows you so well, loves you, and whom you can count on. And in addition to this work that happens in the hypnosis chair, I am going to give you homework. Every single time you find yourself automatically reaching for a cigarette, I'm going to have you to immediately tell yourself *STOP!* and we will identify another physical response for you that will be accompanied by a thought, an internal experience that you will very consciously use to help carve a new pathway in your brain. It is absolutely imperative that you go through this process we create *every single time* you have this feeling that you are going to reach for a cigarette—whether you are *actually* doing it or even just thinking about *maybe* doing it. By making this change, you are in effect *not* going down that old pathway in your brain. You are stopping at the *STOP* sign and going another way. In a short time, that new way will be the easier of the two, and when the original path does not get used, just like an unused path in the forest, it disappears.

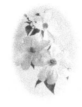

Chapter 8

Forgiveness

Forgiveness is an essential step in releasing subconscious emotional pressure. It is so important that I've given it a chapter of its own. Forgiveness is a topic that is very difficult for most people. You may feel there are past or current experiences in your life that are completely unforgivable. You may feel hurt, disrespected, cheated, betrayed, wronged. Your experience may affect your ability to interact with new people and new situations in your life. Your experience may have led you to avoid certain life events or to approach them in an overly cautious and distrustful manner. You may already be aware that an experience earlier in your life has had a negative effect on your current life. Nearly everyone can identify with this scenario. You may have felt wronged in a way that has colored your ability to enjoy subsequent experiences, your ability to trust new people, and your ability to be open to new experiences in your life. You may even feel there are things *you* have done that are unforgivable. If so, rest assured you are not alone. You don't have to keep carrying the weight of this emotional pain. This chapter can help you.

Behind this difficulty to forgive are the painful emotions of anger, bitterness, feelings of betrayal, unfairness, jealousy. It may be hard for you to admit that you carry these feelings with you. More than likely, you may not be consciously aware of carrying these feelings (illustrated in a moment by Laura, regarding her ex-husband Dan). These reactions to past events can take up residence in our minds and hearts, and color the way we look at the world. Being treated unfairly or disrespectfully can lead to anger which may never have been resolved in a healthy manner. It may even have led to misperceptions about us: that we are not worthy, or that there is something wrong with us. Being hurt by someone can make us cautious when considering new relationships. A betrayal on any level can make trusting others very difficult.

There are so many opportunities in life for us to experience anger, which usually has a root in fear. You may respond with instant anger if another driver cuts you off in traffic, but under that anger may be fear—that the driver's erratic behavior might have caused an accident and harm to you and your children in the back seat. Being jilted by a lover can make you initially angry, but under that anger may be the fear that you are not lovable, that you are not good enough, rich enough, smart enough, and that maybe you will have a hard time finding another lover.

This stew of unpleasant and unresolved memories and emotions is not some benign part of your past. It uses energy on a daily basis. Any time you find yourself reciting the details of a past hurt, sharing the story again, you are feeding that old experience and letting it grow inside you. What you give attention to grows in your awareness. Spending time with these unpleasant memories is stressful. This stress has a negative effect on every part of your body and on every aspect of your health. We all know people who are so preoccupied with being wronged in their past that they have little time and attention to give to the present moment. They never seem to be happy or thriving.

What if you could let those old hurts go? What if you could just use past experiences as sources of information about how you want your life to change going forward? What if you thought about your past as compost for your present and future self? How would life be different if you weren't distracted by negative emotions from past hurts? The fact is, most people are not fully aware of all the ways these past experiences have hurt them and colored the way they live their lives. Some things happened so long ago you may not even be able to remember them consciously. But whether you remember them or not, they are there. And from these experiences, you have developed beliefs about yourself and about the world, personality traits, and habits of behavior and thought. These lead to the life you are presently living.

Forgiveness is sometimes described as an antidote to anger. You can probably remember a time, perhaps recently, when you felt angry. Perhaps you were treated unfairly, or someone treated you disrespectfully. Something may have happened that led you to believe you were about to suffer a loss. Remember what that day was like for you? The anger may have been your dominant emotion that day. It overshadowed feelings you might otherwise have had that day, like joy, pleasure, happiness. Anger sucks your energy. Anger unattended can simmer away, and its continued presence can even grow and become more disruptive as, without intending to, you let it grow by continuing to give it attention. As you continue to think about it, it becomes part of your internal soundtrack: what you are thinking about all day. It becomes part of your external soundtrack as you share your life experiences with people around you. This negative energy robs you of your ability to focus on positive aspects of life. It robs you of your ability to enjoy life and to find pleasure and meaning in life. When you have residual anger from wrongs done to you in the past, that causes emotional pressure. This emotional pressure can erupt in all sorts of ways. It can express itself as misperceptions about your own self-worth or lovability, as limiting beliefs or mental thought habits like "I've never been good at/I can't/ I'll never have—" and as physical manifestations, like chronic back pain or migraine headaches.

My client Laura came to me for help with migraine headaches. In the course of our session, I learned that she had an ex-husband named Dan who had lied and cheated and ultimately left her. "I forgave Dan a long time ago," Laura said, waving her hand as if this comment was an inconsequential bit of trivia. She described her new husband and reported feeling happy. But in hypnosis, it was apparent to both of us that she was still suffering from Dan's rejection and from his infidelity, and she was deeply hurt and extremely angry. In hypnosis, she was able to see this clearly and to release her anger at a deeper level. She was able to appreciate the grief she still felt from the loss of that relationship. Recognizing an emotion and putting it into context is the first step toward being able to resolve it and move on in life without residual emotional damage. She was able to review this part of her life in hypnosis, at a subconscious level. She could clearly see how the breakup of her marriage had everything to do with Dan's desire for a different life and little to do with her shortcomings. Although the relationship had been mutually beneficial for many years, a time had come when that was no longer true. She was able to see that it was inevitable that their marriage would need to end. She saw now that it was an advantage for her not to be in that relationship anymore. She acknowledged that her life was more enjoyable and satisfying now. Evaluating this part of her life in hypnosis, where she had access to all of her stored experiences both during that time and since that time, allowed her to see clearly what had happened was better for everyone involved. Then, as we went through the forgiveness process in hypnosis, she found it was easier to *really* forgive him, and she emerged feeling freer, no longer suffering from the feelings of anger and betrayal. Helping her disconnect from that emotional pressure left her feeling lighter. She was able to set down the burden of rejection and disappointment. She was able to set down the constant rumination about believing that she was inadequate and that she had failed in her marriage. I helped her begin her practice of 7th Path Self-Hypnosis®, which reinforced all the work we had done together. She reported sleeping better immediately. Her migraine headaches were infrequent. Her new relationship was personally enriching and she was in the midst of happily changing careers.

Forgiveness of other people doesn't mean you condone what they have done. It does not mean in any way that what they did was acceptable. Forgiveness doesn't mean you are pardoning them or letting them feel like what they did has no consequences, or that it doesn't matter. You will not even be communicating your experience of forgiveness with that person unless you want to.

This process doesn't mean you are forgetting what happened. You do not have to forget what happened. Often there is something valuable to be learned from the situation. Remembering is critical to preventing a similar situation from happening again. Forgiveness does not mean the behavior will be forgotten.

There is no requirement to be open to reconciliation. You may not ever want anything to do with that person. You can keep them excluded from your life in your outer world, and still have privately and silently forgiven them in your internal world. Forgiveness is not even something you share with the person you have forgiven, because it is for you, not for them. It is none of their business unless you choose to share it. You do not have to share your forgiveness with anyone in your life unless you choose to share it.

This gift is for you, not the offender. Forgiveness lets you separate yourself from the pain of the event. It allows you to move on in your life without the heavy load of anger around your neck. It is a way of severing a painful emotional tie. Sometimes in the process of forgiveness in hypnosis, it is helpful to explore reasons that a situation occurred. It can be helpful sometimes, but not always, to explore the motivations and background of the person being forgiven. Sometimes this exploration leads to a greater overall understanding of the situation and decreases the feeling of having been a victim.

I help all my clients feel compassion for themselves. Sometimes clients have assumed some level of responsibility in the situation that is not appropriate given that they were just a child or a young person when the event occurred. It can be helpful to review the event from a perspective of now being older and wiser. Just what was happening back then, and what were the intentions and motivations of the people involved? Often when clients understand that the person they are forgiving was acting in response to events in their life, and not intentionally trying to ruin the life of someone else, it can be easier to forgive them. Again, not to forget, condone, pardon, or reconcile.

Understand the importance of ongoing forgiveness. Forgiveness is a skill, and like any skill, you become more proficient with practice. Sometimes the person you are forgiving is still in your life. Sometimes you may have to still see them, be in the same room with them. Or you may see other people or situations which remind you of him or her. That's when the habit of ongoing forgiveness becomes so valuable to you. Marilyn struggled after forgiving her mother for something that happened earlier in her life. She learned about the value of ongoing forgiveness, and I taught her Object Projection, which I describe in Chapter 11. She goes into the kitchen with her sister and does Cross-Body Swing (also described in Chapter 11.) She uses these powerful techniques when she attends family gatherings several times a year where her mother's presence reminds her of the hurtful behaviors. She is casting a wide net. I encourage you to also do whatever you need to do to help yourself. You need to prepare yourself for the times when you may be reminded of those old feelings, ready with an attitude of ongoing forgiveness to keep yourself emotionally safe and disconnected from the actions of the person you are forgiving.

Malachy McCourt, an Irish American author, once said, "Resentment is like taking poison and expecting the other person to die." The reason you forgive others is to release yourself from pain. Disconnecting yourself with forgiveness from painful past experiences and the negative emotions that accompany them leave you feeling lighter, with much more energy to direct to your present life, and to your future. Disconnecting yourself from this major source of stress can contribute to decreased physical pain of all kinds, including migraines.

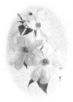

Chapter 9

Self-Sabotage

Sometimes when the therapy process is not having as much of a positive effect as I expect, it is because there is some part of a client's psyche that is getting benefit from not changing.

For example, a young girl came to see me for a consultation by her mother—she was having pain in her right foot. I always require a referral from a doctor before doing hypnosis for the purpose of managing pain. The doctor readily agreed because he felt he had exhausted every possible source of foot pain. He did not believe there was anything wrong with her foot.

It was clear after a very short conversation with the girl and her mother this mother was completely devoted to helping her daughter overcome her foot pain. She had taken time off work to take her daughter to multiple different therapists—her primary doctor, a foot specialist, physical therapist—they had even gone to see a surgeon. They had even traveled to see doctors away from home and spent the night in a hotel together. No one was able to find a specific problem that could be "fixed." It was clear to me immediately that this young girl was receiving a great benefit from all the time and attention her mother was giving her.

Concurrently, the young girl had a lot of doctor notes that gave her days off from sports activities. As a result, she became the equipment manager and record keeper. She got to spend extra time with her teacher because of this.

In hypnosis, I was not surprised to find out that she didn't really like sports where she had to run. She never had. In hypnosis, we found out what she really wanted to do was become an artist. She hadn't been able to talk about this with her family, because they had already decided that she should go to college and get a professional job like other people in her family. And almost everyone in the family was involved with sports. By having foot pain, she received the secondary gain of an excuse not to play sports, and she also enjoyed the extra time with her teacher and her mother. She also got time and attention from doctors, nurses, and therapists. This was a big difference from her home life, where she was one of four children. She also had an excuse not to attend sports events her siblings were involved in (which she privately thought were boring) because there was usually a lot of walking involved to get out to the fields.

In hypnosis, she was able to understand this and became consciously aware of this. Her mother, who had been in attendance at all of the hypnotherapy sessions, was very supportive, enrolling her daughter in an after-school arts program. Both her mother and her father stopped insisting she participate in after-school sports programs.

Understand the role others play in your life regarding migraines. Are there interpersonal interactions that are associated with or precede a migraine? Are you punishing someone else with your migraines? Are your migraines setting up scenarios where someone has to take time off work, or do extra work because you are incapacitated?

Do you need this pain to get attention from someone? This happens sometimes. Sometimes a health crisis in a family can elicit attention and caregiving from other family members. It might be hard to get attention from someone, but when you are suffering, perhaps you get sympathy and offers of help. Suffering can get you attention, and perhaps you don't know another healthier way to get attention.

If there is something you do that will bring on a migraine most of the time, and you still do it anyway, this is worth spending some time thinking about. If you know you are going to get a migraine and you still do that thing, why are you hurting yourself? Is there a hidden value to you for suffering from migraine pain? Do you get extra attention from friends or family members? Are you avoiding something? I'm not saying this is you, but it might be. A migraine is an expensive way to avoid something, but it is an effective way. And remember, our brain likes to do things with the least amount of effort possible. So if you want to avoid something and getting a horrid headache lets you avoid it, wham! Migraine on! Avoidance achieved!

I have a personal story about how I sabotaged myself and locked in a migraine headache as a response to a situation. Alcohol was a key trigger for me with migraines. It didn't take much for me to get a migraine. After even two glasses of wine with dinner, if I didn't keep myself very well hydrated with water, I'd wake up at three a.m. in terrible pain. For years, I was married to a man who liked to drink wine and collect it, to a degree. I love wine, all the varied tastes and how much fun it is to match with different flavors of food. I like the relaxation I feel when I drink wine or other alcoholic beverages. For a while, I thought that alcohol was the main trigger for my migraine headaches. I had so much pain that it kept me from drinking too much or too frequently. Alcoholism runs in my family, and worry about the possibility of becoming an alcoholic myself was always in the back of my mind. I told myself that Mother Nature gave me migraines to prevent me from becoming an alcoholic. In some way, I had accepted at a subconscious level that as long as I had migraine pain, I wouldn't become an alcoholic. I set myself up for pain every single time I drank alcohol.

Self-sabotage is something none of us likes to think we do, but the fact is that it's quite common. You may be unaware of the ways in which you sabotage yourself. An easy example is what happened to Sharon. She wanted to lose weight, but sometimes she also wanted to have a candy bar. When she went to the grocery store, there was a whole aisle devoted to candy. She noticed her favorite candy bar. It came in four ounces, eight ounces, or a bag of "Mini" sizes—thirty small one ounce bars, and they were not much more expensive than a larger bar. She chose the big bag and said to herself that it's a better "deal," and she'll only eat one ounce. But when she got home, it was so easy to eat one after the other. If she'd just bought one small candy bar, taken it home and eaten it mindfully, enjoying it fully, it would have probably satisfied her desire for a candy bar. Instead, she had an entire bag of candy calling her name from the cupboard and she ate candy every day until the bag was empty– many more calories than just one bar. She felt frustrated by this but kept doing it anyway. In hypnosis, we identified that part of her does want to lose weight and to be slim and trim. And we also noticed there was a part of her that wanted to eat as much candy as she wanted and not care about the impact. We did a little exercise where we let each part have her say and let the two parts talk back and forth to one another. As the hypnotist, my job was to be the mediator, to be sure that each part's desire and also their stake in the ultimate outcome—the woman having a happy and satisfying life— was fully expressed and understood by the other.

We isolated *The Part That Wants to Eat as Much Candy* as *I Want to and Not Care About the Impact*. There was another part we named *The Part That Remembers Nothing Tastes as Good as Slender Feels*. We did a lot of inner role play on a subconscious level in hypnosis. We made sure that each part had their time to say how they felt and what they ultimately wanted. We found that *The Part that Wants to Eat as Much Candy as I Want to* also wanted to be slim and trim. We ultimately gave *I Want to Eat as Much Candy as I Want to* a new name and a new role: *Enforcer of The French Woman's 3 Bite Rule*. It was her job to be sure that once a week— she chose Saturdays—she could have three bites of whatever dessert she wanted.

This made all the difference in helping her free herself from compulsively stuffing sweets into her mouth. She stopped buying bags of candy bars at the grocery store. She can have three bites of any dessert she desires, once a week. The first three bites are always the most delicious anyway, and she knows in a week she can do it again if she wants. So *The Part That Wants to Eat as Much Candy as I Want to* accepted this new role that fits in better with the way she really wanted to be in life—slim and trim, feeling attractive. That new part,

Enforcer of The French Woman's 3 Bite Rule makes sure that on the weekly occasions when she does have sweets, it is something special, and is limited to three delicious bites. A few months later, she sent me a note and said her weight was lower than it had been in nine years.

We call this kind of therapy process *Parts Mediation Therapy*. To be clear, this does not mean a client has a personality disorder of any kind or multiple personalities. This is just a way of thinking about inner conflicts, and we all have them. There are parts of us that want to do one thing, and parts of us that want something else.

One of the questions I ask clients before we ever do hypnosis is, "Do you feel like you should be punished for something you once did?" So many people beat themselves up for mistakes they made, or for perceived wrongs they feel responsible for. I ask this question because people can be brutal beyond belief to themselves when they feel guilty for something. If there is something in your life that you feel guilty about, you may be punishing yourself on a regular basis in one way or another. Self-punishment is a type of self-sabotage. And if this is happening, it is very likely to be happening at a subconscious level. Your hypnotherapist can help you change your limiting belief that you deserve to suffer forever. Luckily your subconscious mind is a treasure trove of all the experiences you have ever had and the information you need to change is available to you in hypnosis.

Perhaps there is something you need to do to make a past situation "right." If so, do it, and give yourself the gift of self-esteem that comes from doing the right thing.

Sometimes, however, a sense of responsibility and culpability can be established when you are too young to even be aware of the appropriateness of your emotional response. In hypnosis, I have helped people remember the source of these feelings, and often they are surprised, saying, for example in the case of Willow, *"It wasn't my responsibility to watch my little sister when she had that accident. I was only seven. My mother should have been more attentive."* In the case of Theresa, hypnosis helped her identify the truth about a situation she had taken responsibility for subconsciously in early childhood, leading her to self-soothe in a manner that led to the development of skin-picking behaviors that left her thighs disfigured. *"It wasn't my fault my parents fought and my dad left us. I was only five years old."*

What a relief that can be, to have clarity and to generate insight for yourself. The emotional pressure from these chronic negative feelings, whether conscious or unconscious, contributes to any number of stress-related symptoms, including physical pain, and for some people, migraine headaches.

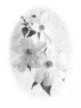

Chapter 10

New Patterns for a Pain-Free Life—
Setting Yourself up for Success

"If you always do what you've always done, you'll always get what you always got."

– Henry Ford & **Tony Robbins**

Culturing awareness of your internal "state" and your internal "soundtrack" is an important skill to develop. Many of us were brought up with the expectation that we would feel and do and be what other people expected of us. Being aware of how you feel in any given moment is the first step in gaining sovereignty in your life. You do not need to be at the mercy of situations and events and other people in your life.

Your primary responsibility is to take care of yourself first. If you are caring well for yourself, you can live very intentionally, headache free. Then you have the ability to care well for people and things in your life that are important to you.

Changing Your "State"

"State Changing" is a valuable skill that few people possess, and it is worth cultivating. "State Changing" is the ability to notice exactly how you feel in the moment, and then *change* it. It is having the skill to notice and access practiced strategies for immediate relief in the moment. Being able to *notice* how you feel at any moment and *change* how you feel is something you can learn. You can learn this outside of hypnosis. These tools are even more effective if taught and rehearsed in hypnosis. I teach stress reduction tools to every single client. I have described them in the next chapter. I want you to master these. They are the key to changing your internal experience in life. No one likes to feel out of control, angry, irritated, frustrated. These emotions can be exhausting. This is an important part of the plan to help you eliminate migraine headaches. Remember, I told you this was a multi-pronged approach, and we are casting a wide net. These will help you in everyday situations, and have other positive side ripples, helping you feel calm and centered and in control and not at the mercy of your feelings or outside events.

Changing Your "Soundtrack"

Changing your "soundtrack." You spend vastly more time with yourself than with anyone else. Yet many people have a negative soundtrack in their mind all the time. Notice yours. What are you saying to yourself about yourself throughout the day? Are you an enthusiastic champion, a best friend to yourself? Or are you saying things to yourself that you would never say out loud to anyone else? Your internal soundtrack has more of a role in your life experience than you realize. Because of the way our subconscious mind works, if you tell yourself something over and over, after a while you start to believe it. A belief is just a thought you think over and over again. With this understanding, it is critical that the soundtrack in your head be positive.

I learned this decades ago, on my knees in the butterfly garden at the Skagit Valley Master Gardener's two-acre demonstration garden in Washington State. All of the new Master Gardeners volunteered in the demonstration garden, and I was there on a cloudy afternoon with my new Master Gardener friend Maggie. We were on our hands and knees, weeding. I don't remember what I said that day out loud, about myself, but I remember the way it made me feel. It was something mean. And Maggie sat back on her heels and said, "Kathie! Don't ever say that about yourself! You would never say that out loud to a friend!" And she was right. And it brought me an awareness of my internal soundtrack.

My mother brought this home to me again some years later. We had paused on the stairs of my new home to look at some of the family photos I'd collected on the walls there. We were focused on a beautiful photo of my mother, taken the day she turned fifteen, her hair shiny, her skin glowing with that fresh budding beauty that young women have. She had a single pearl on a chain around her neck. "I felt so ugly that day," she told me. I looked at her incredulously. It was a beautiful picture of a beautiful young woman. "I know." She nodded with a sad sigh, looking at the picture nostalgically. Then she turned to me and said, "Don't do that to yourself, Kathie. I hope you are not doing that to yourself." And I realized I *was*. I was privately telling myself every day I wasn't pretty enough, thin enough, organized enough, clever enough. And I took a good look at my life and this lesson from my mother, and I changed how I talked to myself every day. And this time, it stuck.

Use affirmations to help you keep your internal soundtrack positive. Affirmations are one of the seven ways that the 7th Path® Recognitions can be used. These affirmations help you stay focused on positive truths about yourself and about your intentions.

You will know you have changed your internal soundtrack successfully when you notice a more positive and optimistic outlook, and when the story you tell yourself and others is less about suffering and being a victim of external forces (other people and situations, including migraine pain) and more about surviving, thriving, and happiness and joy in the moment.

People sometimes ask, "What is the difference between meditation and self-hypnosis?" Before I learned 7th Path Self-Hypnosis®, I tried a formal meditation practice, first at the Buddhist Center in Bellingham, Washington, and then with the help of a wonderful mindfulness counselor. I was just not able to sit in stillness for twenty minutes at a time. I tried, and I couldn't do it. For me, 7th Path Self-Hypnosis® was something I could do easily. In 7th Path Self-Hypnosis®, developed by Cal Banyan, there are nine "Recognitions" which are given to you in hypnosis. There are seven different ways to use them, hence the name 7th Path. The Recognitions are pearls of wisdom, and something you learn inside the class, while in hypnosis. In both traditional meditation and in 7th Path Self-Hypnosis®, you are sending yourself into a quieter brainwave state, opening yourself up for calm centeredness and insight. 7th Path Self-Hypnosis® leads you to a state of being suggestible, and one of the ways you use the nine Recognitions is as hypnotic suggestions. 7th Path Self-Hypnosis® also works to maintain the gains made from the 5-PATH® hypnotherapy process. You will know you're doing it right when it bothers you if you miss a session.

7th Path Self-Hypnosis® enables you to live your life in a way that keeps you feeling positive and engaged.

Regular practice sets you up for fresh insights and for calm centeredness that follows you into the rest of your day. In my case, doing 7th Path Self-Hypnosis® before bed has led to better sleep, fewer bad dreams, and fewer migraines.

Remember to continue to manage your external triggers. Managing these triggers requires vigilance, but it gets easier every day. Once you give yourself the gift of 5-PATH® Hypnosis and you no longer have emotional pressure from your past, from mistaken perceptions and limiting beliefs, you have a lot more energy for everything else in your life.

I encourage my clients to practice 7th Path Self-Hypnosis® twice a day, for twenty minutes each time. Practicing 7th Path Self-Hypnosis® daily can also help you learn to relax, and can help you be more focused and improve your concentration. Learn and use the tools in the De-Stress Kit in the next chapter. Choose to make space in your life for self-care. You need to say no to outside requests in order to have time and energy to say yes to yourself.

If you are curious about the mechanics of hypnosis, go to hypnosis school. Erika Flint of Cascade Hypnosis Center in Bellingham, WA is booked out months for her classes, but she is an excellent instructor and worth waiting for. There are other 5-PATH® instructors and you can find a listing at www.5-PATH.com.

5-PATH® is an insight-based process. I don't know what the answers are for you, for your life. I work with my clients to understand what their needs are and what their goals are.

My job is to be a coach and a guide, to assist you into a hypnotic state where the suggestions and the learning can make a difference.

Listen to your Hypnotherapist's pre-recorded relaxation MP3s. You will learn to relax to the timbre and cadence of your hypnotist's voice. You will go into hypnosis deeper and faster, like going to sleep with a familiar bedtime story.

Be on time, rested, and ready. Hypnosis takes effort. It is not something I do "to" you, it is something we do together. So pave the way for your success—plan ahead and allow time. Be sure to allow time afterward, too, for integration—plan a quiet evening so you don't have a lot of things that need your attention.

Do your homework! There isn't a lot of homework, but there is some, especially at first when you are making a behavior change.

Learn and practice 7th Path Self-Hypnosis®. Any 5-Path Hypnotherapist can teach you 7th PATH Self-Hypnosis®. You can get an app for your phone with bells that you set at intervals to assist you in your practice of the 9 Recognitions.

The basic Recognitions, one through five, are often included in a 5-PATH® Hypnotherapy process. The advanced Recognitions, six through nine, have a more spiritual basis and work with any spiritual orientation or religious belief system. You will learn them while in hypnosis. Again, the Recognitions are small bits of wisdom. They act as positive suggestions to yourself, and because you practice by giving them to yourself while practicing self-hypnosis, they are more powerful than traditional affirmations. They keep your mind focused on positive, basic truths rather than on old mistaken beliefs and misperceptions.

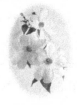

Chapter 11

De-Stress Kit

I have a gift for you. It's a De-Stress kit of seven easy-to-learn techniques I've collected that can help you change your feeling "state" at any moment. All the techniques here have been personally tested (and used!) by me and many of my clients.

These tools work. I teach them regularly to my private clients and in my classes. Culture awareness of your internal "state" and "soundtrack." I want you to learn sovereignty over your feeling state. These state-changing strategies work so well. They give you immediate relief in the moment, are easy to learn, and they take about two minutes each to do. Everyone can benefit from being able to adjust their own "state" when they want to.

I want you to be able to quickly pull out a tool that works for you and to use it immediately, with good results. You'll feel better immediately when you use these. You'll feel better in the moment, and in the future, because you'll know that you have learned a technique that changes how you feel. The more you use these tools, the easier it is to use them and the faster you feel relief, and the faster you feel a calm sense of being in control.

The starting place is noticing. On a scale of one to ten, with ten feeling completely out of control or upset and one feeling calm, centered, peaceful—how do you feel right now? Notice this number. If this feeling had a color, what color would it be? Does it have a shape or a texture? Notice this. Then do one of the techniques. Notice again where you are on the one-to-ten scale.

The Three-Breath Hypnosis Technique

I originally learned this as "The 2 Breath Hypnosis Technique" from Erika Flint, but I have since modified it by observing the natural world, specifically my cat, Magellan. I noticed that when he feels threatened he starts "huffing," doing short, forceful exhales accompanied by a huffing sound, and that reminded me of a public speaking trick I learned years ago. One of the difficulties of talking when we are nervous or upset is that we tense up and tend to breathe shallowly. Breathing shallowly allows carbon dioxide to build up in our blood and makes us feel breathless, like we can't even get a good gulp of air. This has probably happened to you at some time or another. It's very uncomfortable. You may feel like you can't quite catch your breath. It's very hard to relax when you can't catch your breath. Your voice doesn't sound normal, and you and everyone around you can hear that you are nervous. The trick is to start this technique with a good, forceful exhale. Just try that. Try it now. It's kind of like re-setting your breathing. A good, satisfying exhale. A complete exhale. Get rid of that carbon dioxide. If you are alone, you might accompany it with a huffing sound. Make it noisy, for practice. By exhaling forcefully and completely, you make room for the next lungful of oxygen-rich air. Then take that deep, satisfying breath. Think about the fact that the air is rich with oxygen—exactly what your body needs in this moment. Let that breath be deep, pushing through your diaphragm and into your belly. A deep belly breath. Breathing deeply into your belly is important because that tugs on your Vagus nerve, initiating a relaxation response in your body. The relaxation response actually slows your heart rate and lowers your blood pressure, helping you feel calmer and more relaxed.

As you exhale, let it be slow and even. Again, your goal is to get as much carbon dioxide-laden air out of your body as possible. Pause for just a moment, listening to your body.

Wait. You will feel when your body desires a deep breath. As you breathe in, notice how absolutely delicious that breath feels. Repeat the slow and deep inhale, and a slow and thorough exhale. Now you are ready for the next layer to this technique. Do this exercise again, and this time as you breathe out, breathe out that stress color and feel it leaving your body. When you breathe in slowly, you might want to breathe in another color, something that symbolizes relaxation to you. As you breathe out, everything you don't need is leaving your body.

So here's the technique:

1. Breathe out forcefully and completely (think of a pissed-off cat huffing). Really empty your lungs.

2. Take a deep breath of the oxygen-rich air that is all around you, pulling it deep into your lungs, past your diaphragm and into your belly. Let your exhale be slow and steady and complete. As you exhale, exhale all the worry and tension and stress. Exhale the color that reminds you of stress.

3. Repeat: Take a deep breath of the oxygen-rich air that is all around you, pulling it deep into your lungs, past your diaphragm and into your belly. Let your exhale be slow and steady and complete. As you exhale, exhale all the worry and tension and stress. Exhale the color that reminds you of stress.

Now notice what number you are, on the scale of one to ten. How many points did you change? If you went down even one point, note how that entire exercise took all of ninety seconds. Do it again. Now, where are you on the one-to-ten scale?

You just changed your "state" with your breath. You can do this anytime you feel upset or tense. Do it today three times, whether you feel upset and tense or not.

This is also a secret antidote to performance anxiety.

Cross-Body Swing

Cross-body swing. I learned this from Melissa Tiers. She is the originator of this pleasant and effective self-calming technique. Again, note how you feel before you start and give yourself a number on the one-to-ten scale. Stand with your feet shoulder width apart. You'll need something, like a small ball, to pass back and forth, from one hand to the other. Each time you transfer the ball from your right hand to your left hand, you let your right hand cross the midpoint of your body first. Crossing the midpoint of the body causes the two different hemispheres of your brain to work together. This has a calming effect on your brain. Set up a comfortable rhythm. This is pleasant and you can do it while conversing with someone and they will never even know you are using a "State-Changing" stress reduction tool.

Peripheral Vision

This is another tool from Melissa Tiers. I love this technique. I use it all the time. I used it this morning at the grocery store when I had to wait a long time in line and found myself feeling impatient. Again, rate yourself on the one-to-ten scale. Then find a spot to focus on—it could be a spot on the wall. I used a curl in the hair of the woman in line in front of me. Look pointedly at the spot. Now let your gaze soften, and your eyes relax. While you are looking right at that spot, allow your peripheral vision to notice the space in about a 3" circle around the spot. Now without letting your eyes move from the one spot, let yourself become aware of the space in every direction about twelve inches away from that spot. Now allow your awareness to expand to the sides and to the walls of the room. While never taking your eyes off that spot, now let your awareness take in the space above, to the ceiling and below, to the floor. Now let your awareness extend outside of the room up into the sky, and below your feet. It is impossible to return your vision to the focused "eagle eye" concentration that is part of our fight, flight, or freeze response when you soften your gaze. Softening your gaze relaxed your mind. Allow your breathing to be slow and deep during this exercise. Notice your number on the one-to-ten scale. If you came down even one point, that was a ten percent improvement in about three minutes! Pick another spot and do it again, if you like.

Object Projection

Object Projection is so powerful. I use it to help clients deal with unpleasant people or situations in their lives, and with unpleasant habits like smoking, and with fears, like fear of snakes. We'll practice it with a headache. Here's how it works. Notice where you are on the one-to-ten scale. With your eyes closed, note the discomfort in your head. It is like a ball of energy. What color is it? Does it have a texture? Is it sharp and pokey or thick or sticky? Now imagine that you are pulling that feeling, that color, and texture right out of your head and into a ball in front of your chest. Imagine that the ball is about the size of a basketball. Hold that ball of colored energy and squeeze it until it is the size a baseball. Now send that ball out in front of you about three feet. Now bring it back and let it expand back to basketball size. Make the pain and the worry worse. Can you do that? Now make it small again. Push it in your mind out to arm's length again. Now push it out ten feet. Now thirty feet. Now the length of the football field. Manipulating energy can feel very powerful, and this is an effective technique for many things. It can help with pain or anxious feelings. Try it today when a person or situation annoys you. Note afterward what number you are on the one-to-ten scale.

Mental Rehearsal

Mental Rehearsal is a valuable technique used by speakers, musicians, athletes, and you! I learned it from my harp teacher, Harper Tasche, in Seattle, twenty years ago. It's a simple matter of imagining yourself doing something. The trick is to engage all of your senses and to engage your emotions. Say there is a tense situation at work involving you, and there is going to be a meeting about it. First, imagine feeling the way you want you feel. Imagine the absolute best outcome. Really allow the feelings and sensations of that outcome to sink in. Now back up, perhaps to the moments before you enter the meeting room. Imagine walking down the hall, feeling confident. Notice your posture. Notice the relaxed expression on your face. Let your shoulders and neck be loose. Take a slow and comfortable deep breath. Notice how that relaxes your body. Feel yourself mentally composed. Imagine standing at the door, on time and well-prepared. Before you even walk in, imagine that your relaxed and positive demeanor influences everyone the room. Make this real for your brain. How does the hallway smell? How does the doorknob feel? What does the conversation sound like as you enter the room? Now imagine stepping into the room. Imagine yourself smiling, having eye contact, feeling respectful of the other people. Now imagine stepping into the room and changing the tone just by your presence. Imagine sending goodwill to every person in the room silently, modeling for them your peaceful intention to contribute to the highest good for all. Think, "I'm going to feel and be like this, or something better." Let your subconscious mind take it up a notch for you. You can do this a week in advance, the night before, or a few moments in the hallway before stepping into the room, or all three. When you intentionally plan to have an event go well, you are setting yourself up for success. Your subconscious mind will follow your lead. Try it.

Next Smallest Thing

Next Smallest Thing: Thank you again, to Melissa Tiers. I love this technique. It's so wonderful when you are overwhelmed to grab this technique. What tiny step will give you forward momentum? I use this all day to keep me from being overwhelmed. Just do one thing. If you are completely overwhelmed it can be helpful to just jot down everything that you can think of that needs doing, just to get it out of your head. You won't lose it or forget something important, because it is written down. But letting your head have a break from holding onto everything can be a tremendous relief. And then you can look at your list and find the smallest possible step that will give you forward momentum.

Thought-Stopping

Every time I have a client who is trying to do something different, thought-stopping is the first homework assignment they get from me. The 5-PATH® Hypnotherapy process is where the reasons and the root of the problem are uncovered and eliminated, but meanwhile, clients have a habit in their mind that needs to change.

Nail-biting is an easy example. This is what I tell my nail-biting clients: We are going to use your subconscious mind to help you identify and eliminate the thoughts and feelings that led to nail-biting in the first place by using the 5-PATH® Hypnotherapy process. Simultaneously, we need to give your mind an alternative behavior. For probably years, you have bitten your nails. You have done this so many times, so automatically, that it is the path of least resistance for your brain. You feel uncomfortable in some way, and your automatic response is to bite your nails. From now on, every time you find yourself biting your nails, or every time you become aware of the feeling of wanting to bite your nails you are going to say STOP! to yourself, inside your head. We want to put up a big roadblock on that neural pathway in your brain. It is a comfortable, easy path because you have gone down that path so many times. It's automatic in your brain. We need to eliminate that path once and for all. So starting right now, you are not to go down that path. Not even one more time. The minute you catch yourself biting or wanting to bite, you say STOP! and you put your thumb and index finger together on each hand. This gives your fingers something else to do, and it serves as an anchor for this behavior change that you are helping your brain accomplish. At the same time, I have people identify the feeling and color and shape of their unhappiness with this habit, bringing all the embarrassment and shame and discomfort that goes along with nail-biting into their chest, really trying to feel it, as bad as it ever gets. I coach them to let that unhappy color drain out of their body, through the soles of their feet, as if that color was being magnetized down into the earth. That unpleasant energy will quickly be absorbed into the earth, and be recycled into something beautiful somewhere else. The important thing is that the client says to themselves STOP! and immediately visualizes the unpleasant color draining quickly out through the soles of their feet. Sometimes clients like to feel the unpleasant color replaced with another calmer color, and this might be warmer or cooler—whatever feels to the client like relief and self-control and peacefulness. I have clients practice this during hypnosis, while they are in an Alpha brainwave state. It is even more effective when practiced during hypnosis. I have them practice again immediately upon emerging from hypnosis and here is the homework: Say STOP! and do the full color/feeling draining exercise. Do this every single time that the urge to bite your nails occurs. For some clients, this might be dozens of time a day or hundreds of times in a week. Usually, if my instructions are followed, there is relief in a matter of days. The problem is almost always decreased by fifty percent in the first week. It is absolutely essential that this homework is done one hundred percent of the time. It can be a lot of work. We do not want your brain to go back down that neural pathway of feeling uncomfortable and biting one more time. Not one. Every single time, you want to give it a new pathway, and in a very short period, usually days or at most a few weeks, the new pathway becomes the more familiar pathway and the old pathway, no longer used, becomes, using the path in the forest analogy, overgrown and hard to even see. Those connections from nerve cell to nerve cell that used to respond automatically to even the slightest discomfort by compelling you to put your fingers in your mouth and bite your nails are no longer getting oxygenated, and the connections between the cells atrophy, and then this pathway no longer feels satisfying. Meanwhile, the root causes of the original behavior are being discovered and managed by the hypnotherapy process. This part of the process is happening at the subconscious level. The identification and resolution of the problem or problems that are at the root of the nail-biting have to be identified and there has to be a resolution at the subconscious level. Then conscious work can be done to do the homework over and over. One will not work without the other. Both of these must be done together—identifying the very beginning of the problem, which is in your subconscious mind and then deliberately creating a new way of responding to the uncomfortable feeling.

I have shown you specific things you can do to change the way you feel. Remember always to follow up each technique by re-assessing where you are on the one-to-ten scale. If anyone of these brings you down a point on the ten-point scale, you have just decreased your sensation of stress by ten percent. Do it again. That took all of two minutes. Do it again. Try another tool. You have more power than you realize to change your state. State changing is an immensely valuable skill. With practice, these techniques become instantaneous, and with time, effortless. You will be able to literally change your state in seconds. I often practice these with my clients at the beginning and end of hypnosis sessions. I want you to be able to use these anytime and to be able to remember them easily. They work.

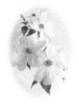

Chapter 12

Barriers

I understand there are challenges in following this path to migraine relief. Giving yourself permission to take care of yourself is the first step, and this is very hard for some people, especially if you are someone accustomed to putting other people's needs first. You may be very, very good at taking care of other people, and not so good at taking care of yourself.

You may not know anyone personally who has benefited from hypnosis. It can feel like taking a big chance to do something new and unfamiliar. If this is the case, then I hope this book has answered some of your questions and helped you realize how effective hypnosis is, and how anyone can benefit from it.

It's important in life to make deliberate choices. As you look back on your life, how many decisions and forks in the road of your life were deliberate choices versus things just "happening?" You have the ability to be in the driver's seat of your life. Go where you want instead of where the wind blows you. Choose to do something that improves your life. Remember, a different approach leads to a different outcome.

It can be hard to do this process alone. You can review all the self-care points here and employ them, but the hypnosis needs a hypnotist. I recommend you find a 5-PATH® Hypnotherapist (www.5-path.com). 7th Path Self-Hypnosis® works best paired with 5-PATH® Hypnosis, because the Recognitions, or hypnotic suggestions, come directly out of the 5-PATH® therapy process. You can order a book and CD set to teach you the basic recognitions of 7th Path Self-Hypnosis®, but it is much more effective if you learn directly from a 7th Path teacher. If you do 5-PATH® Hypnosis with a 5-PATH® Hypnotherapist, he or she can teach you all 9 Recognitions, both the basic and the advanced. This is the best way to get the absolute most out of hypnosis for eliminating migraine headache pain. 5-PATH® Hypnotherapists have some of the most advanced training available. 5-PATH® is an insight-based process that generates self-knowledge and self-understanding. 7th Path Self-Hypnosis® is designed to go hand in hand with 5-PATH® Hypnosis. It is more effective if learned in the context of 5-PATH®. It is deeply meaningful if practiced on a regular basis. Ideally, 7th Path Self-Hypnosis® is practiced for twenty minutes twice a day. Many people spend more time than that looking at their computer and phone screens each day without noticeable improvement in the quality of their lives.

Finally, as much as I would like to say I have a fail-proof magic hypnosis wand, I don't. So, when the occasional migraine sneaks in past your careful efforts at prevention, remember not to fight it. Fighting makes everything worse. Float it– just float through it, use all the pain management options you have—medications, hot/cold therapy, environmental adjustments—and don't beat yourself up. Don't use that time to try to analyze what went wrong. Just be ruthlessly compassionate for yourself in the moment, and remember that pain is temporary. There will be time later to sort things out, to figure out what strategies you can employ more intensively to be more successful in preventing the next migraine headache. This is a complicated business. Cut yourself some slack. Keep your focus on the positive, and continue doing all the things that have been helping you.

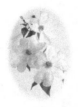

Chapter 13

Conclusion

Migraine headaches are not in charge of your life. You are in charge of your life. Put yourself first, so you have the energy for yourself and for the people and things you care about. As Mary Oliver wrote: "What are you going do with your one wild and precious life?"

As I shared with you, I have a lot of personal experience struggling with and suffering from migraine pain. In my case, I came to hypnosis as a client to sleep better and to work through my procrastination so I could finish some creative projects. For me, migraine pain relief was a side-effect of the 5-PATH® Hypnotherapy process and my daily practice of 7th Path Self-Hypnosis®. This exemplifies an important concept: A positive change in any important area of your life can have a ripple effect beyond what you intend, improving other aspects of your life experience. And this is particularly true when the positive changes are brought about at a subconscious level in hypnosis. Deep introspection and compassion for yourself and others, gained by insight at a subconscious level, smooths the way for a richly rewarding life experience.

My personal experience with pain relief has changed my hypnosis practice. I am more committed to helping my clients adopt the regular practice of 7th Path Self-Hypnosis®. While any meditation practices are likely to benefit you, 7th Path Self-Hypnosis® is easier to learn and to practice, and the statements, or Recognitions, that you say to yourself act as suggestions to your subconscious mind. You are seeding your subconscious mind with positivity and self-acceptance twice a day. If you practice daily, you will experience positive change in your life. It's inevitable.

One of my favorite client stories is Frank. He came to see me after I helped his wife with another problem. Frank had a story much like mine—decades of migraine pain. He'd seen some of the same practitioners I had over the years—he'd also tried nearly everything. He didn't have any experience with any kind of meditation practice, but I started him out listening to my MP3 recording at home, so he got used to the feeling of being awake and deeply relaxed with his mind focused. That was a good segue way to learning 7th Path. He started out, like all my clients, practicing 7th Path Self-Hypnosis twice a day for five minutes. Each week he increased the time by five minutes until he was practicing self-hypnosis for twenty minutes at a time, twice a day. At first, he didn't think he could put himself into self-hypnosis, but I showed him how easy it was during our second session together. Every week we reviewed how his daily progress was going. He told me after just the first month of regular practice that he was already noticing a decrease in his headaches. Three months later, he reported that his migraines are rare, instead of frequent, he has more energy, and he was enjoying the extra time he had now that he wasn't losing time to headache pain. He was practicing 7th Path Self-Hypnosis® regularly and noticed that he also felt calmer and happier. This is very common in new practitioners of 7th Path Self-Hypnosis®. He told me he'd started taking golf lessons, something he'd always wanted to do.

Hypnosis changed my daily experience of life. In addition to migraine relief, sleeping better, and leaving nonstop nightmares behind, I've been able to finish big creative projects like this book. I gained insight about myself, how I came to be the person I am. I gained more compassion for myself in the process, and I am more generous to myself now. The subconscious and conscious processes of letting go of negative feelings have allowed me to feel more relaxed about everything in my life. I just don't feel stressed like I used to. Most importantly, I learned that practicing 7th Path Self-Hypnosis® twice a day is a migraine preventer for me.

Hypnosis works so well because it allows you to reach your subconscious mind, and as I described earlier, your subconscious mind has a bigger role in your life experience than you probably realized. Your subconscious mind is in control of much of your life, not your conscious mind.

Outside triggers for migraine pain can be consciously managed, but nearly all of us could do a better job. Remembering what we want is the first step. Then it is easier, when we are making decisions, to make choices that lead us away from pain. Of course, everyone would prefer to be pain free. You've no doubt identified things you can do better to decrease your migraine pain.

Inside triggers to pain are complex, and that idea is a new concept to many people. Your subconscious mind is an amazing memory bank where you have stored difficult experiences, unresolved emotions, and the beliefs and perceptions that your brain assigned to those events and relationships in every period of your life. Some of those beliefs are self-limiting. Some of those perceptions are mistaken. These deep-seated feelings about yourself hold you back and may be contributing to pain.

You do not have the ability to remember every significant event in your life. You simply don't have conscious access to all the experiences that have contributed to emotional distress in your subconscious. Inner conflicts contribute to emotional pressure. Subconscious emotional pressure from unresolved or painful events and memories surface in our lives as unwanted behaviors, negative or disruptive thoughts, distressing feelings, and physical problems like pain. Sorting out these difficult or painful memories and examining them in the light of our adult perspective is something easily accomplished with 5-PATH® Hypnosis. It doesn't even take a lot of time. It is not necessary to review each and every event in your life to have a helpful outcome. Your subconscious mind has the ability to extrapolate understanding across experiences and across memories. 5-PATH® Hypnosis can be thought of as a rapid change therapy—certainly more rapid than traditional talk therapy which happens at a conscious level.

You may not have conscious awareness of the sources of emotional pressure in your life. You may be aware of the effects in your life because that emotional pressure manifests in your body as troublesome patterns of behavior, "bad habits;" unpleasant feelings; negative patterns of thought, such as "I'm not…, I can't…, I'll never be able to…;" or as pain.

Forgiveness plays an important role in changing habits of behavior, habits of thought, and habits of feeling, and in managing pain and other disabilities that result from emotional distress. And you can't always consciously identify who in your life is causing the most stress at a subconscious level. Many times, clients are surprised during this part of the therapy process. Then they get to feel the immediate relief that comes from disconnecting from that pain and the fresh energy they have in their lives because they are not having to spend energy deep inside themselves managing their subconscious anger about someone.

Self-sabotage happens sometimes. None of us like to think we'd sabotage ourselves, yet there can be many reasons this occurs. I gave you an example in that chapter from my own life. And I spent time on encouraging you to become aware of your internal "state" and your "internal soundtrack" and how to intentionally guide your feelings and thoughts. This is critically important. To help with that, I included a chapter on de-stressing techniques, most of which I learned from Melissa Tiers, author of The Anti-Anxiety Toolkit: Rapid Techniques to Rewire the Brain, and several other books. I've included the techniques I find most helpful for myself and for my clients.

Your subconscious mind has the answers you need. Accessing it can be difficult, but this is what hypnosis is good for—accessing emotions and giving past experiences the benefit of our older, wiser perspectives. We emerge with a deep understanding and compassion, and the emotional pressure is released.

While hypnosis may not be the answer for everyone, for many people it can be part of the answer. It's helpful for so many problems because so many problems have the same root—deep, subconscious misperceptions of difficult or even everyday events, and mistaken beliefs that are damaging to our feelings of self-worth. Emotional tension often expresses itself in the body as pain. Carrying emotional tension and experiencing the subconscious pressure of that tension daily is just exhausting. Gaining insight, or bits of wisdom, from your own experience of being connected with your subconscious mind has positive effects that ripple out into every part of your life. In my experience, most people report benefits beyond what they came to me for. In my case, the extra benefit was migraine relief.

Life can be even better than you imagine. Living without regular migraine pain can open up your life to all sorts of possibilities. This happened to me, and I have seen it repeatedly in my clients. I wish this for you, as well.

On my website, www.SalishSeaHypnosis.com, I have a free MP3 "Relaxation" which I recorded that you are welcome to download and use. If you're ready to live your life migraine-free, then I invite you to contact me at info@ SalishSeaHypnosis.com so we can continue your journey together!

Acknowledgements

To my Journaling Group: the five of us have met every two weeks for over ten years: Carolyn Koehnline, Joan Wildfield, Laura Shelton, Claudia Ackerman.

Tom Ensign, for taking me to the party where I met Tracy Gray.

Tracy Gray, for inspiring me with her party hypnosis and for telling me that people can be helped to quit smoking in as little as one to two sessions.

Jami Engholm, for giving me a year-long education at Bellingham Technical College in her Hypnosis and Hypnotherapy program. I was well prepared to go on to 5-PATH®.

Erika Flint, for giving me my first amazing experience as a client in hypnosis, for her skilled teaching of the 5-PATH® and 7th Path Self-Hypnosis® programs, and for her ongoing mentorship.

Cal Banyan, for developing 5-PATH® Hypnosis and 7th Path Self-Hypnosis®, for writing and teaching The Secret Language of Feelings, and for his support and encouragement.

Elsom Eldridge, for encouraging me to write a book to help other people.

My daughters, Tanya Hanlon and Amy Hanlon, and my sister Lee Todd.

Thanks to my book Launch Team: Tamara Sterling, Stephe Newell Niggemeyer, Brenda Titus, Lynne Potter Lord, Amanda Troy, Paulette Deckers, Marcella Hilferty, and Denise Aguilar.

A special thank you to Angela Lauria of The Author Incubator for her mentorship and support: this book would never have been written without her.

To the Morgan James Publishing team: Special thanks to David Hancock, CEO & Founder for believing in me and my message. To my Author Relations Manager, Margo Toulouse, thanks for making the process seamless and easy. Many more thanks to everyone else, but especially Jim Howard, Bethany Marshall, and Nickcole Watkins.

About the Author

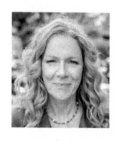Kathie Hardy is a 5-PATH® Hypno-therapist and 7th Path Self-Hypnosis® Instructor with a private practice in Bellingham, WA. She left a successful career in nursing administration and in bedside nursing in ICUs and Emergency Departments after realizing the impact hypnosis can have in helping people overcome addictions, change habits and behaviors, and manage pain. Kathie's lifelong struggle with migraine headaches and her experience both being hypnotized and helping clients with hypnosis make her the perfect person to walk you through the process of evaluating

whether or not hypnosis is right for you. Kathie plays Celtic Harp professionally, and is an avid downhill skier and Master Gardener.